Pre-Medicated Murder?

Other books

By Leland Cooley (Member, Authors League of America):
THE RUN FOR HOME
GOD'S HIGH TABLE
THE RICHEST POOR FOLKS
THE TROUBLE WITH HEAVEN
CONDITION PINK
CALIFORNIA

By Leland Cooley and Lee Cooley:
THE SIMPLE TRUTH ABOUT WESTERN LAND INVESTMENT
THE RETIREMENT TRAP
HOW TO AVOID THE RETIREMENT TRAP
LAND INVESTMENT, USA

Leland Cooley and
Lee Morrison Cooley

PRE-MEDICATED MURDER?

Your Self-Defense Manual

CHILTON BOOK COMPANY   Radnor, Pennsylvania

Copyright © 1974 by Leland Frederick Cooley and Lee Morrison
Cooley
First Edition   *All Rights Reserved*
Published in Radnor, Pa., by Chilton Book Company
and simultaneously in Ontario, Canada
by Thomas Nelson & Sons, Ltd.
Manufactured in the United States of America
Designed by Adrianne Onderdonk Dudden

LIBRARY OF CONGRESS CATALOGING IN PUBLICATION DATA

Cooley, Leland Frederick.
  Pre-medicated murder?

  1. Drugs—Physiological effect.   2. Drug abuse.
3. Drugs—Toxicology.   I. Cooley, Lee Morrison, joint
author.   II. Title.
RM301.C62   1974   614.3'5'0973   74-10674
ISBN 0-8019-5917-9

This book is for
H. MARK YOUNG, M.D., *La Jolla, California,*
and
MURRAY HOFFSTEIN, M.D., *New York City,*
without whose skill and responsibleness one half
of this collaboration would not have been possible,
and for which the "other half" is eternally grateful!

Contents

Nota Bene!

Because modern medicine is so expensive, it has been said that "death is the poor man's only doctor." With all of the great charitable clinics and city, county and state medical facilities, that is not entirely true. Perhaps it would have been more accurate to say that "pre-mature death is the unaware person's only doctor"; for surely with great facilities, with great medical institutions whose trained personnel are available to the very poor, there is no reason for those who need it most and can least afford it to go unattended.

That is not to say that American medical services are even marginally perfect, for they are not. Neither are they ever likely to be, in a free enterprise society. Surely, as we have seen from reports abroad, socialized medicine is not the answer. Nor is medicine as practiced in the socialist Iron Curtain countries where people are regarded as "human work machines" who are evaluated on the number of productive units they contribute to the economy.

Probably, there will never be a time when our health maintenance system is perfect. Certainly there will never be a time when it is not *better than it was.* And positively, there will never be a time when every person in the land does absolutely everything that should be done to ensure optimum health. The problem? The vagaries of human nature.

Unlimited fear and limited finances cause a good part of the trouble. The very wealthy can indulge their fears and insecurities as often as their physicians, surgeons and psychiatrists can see them. The very poor can wait—often too long—in the corridors of overcrowded public facilities where overworked doctors and nurses do the best they can. But it is the not-so-rich and the not-so-poor—members of the families in the middle strata of our economy—who most often become the victims of their own poor judgment where health treatment and maintenance are concerned.

Sometimes as we (the authors) went about gathering material for this work, we had the feeling that our pioneer forebears may have been better off in so far as self-diagnosis and medication were concerned.

We do not speak of those serious diseases they called "brain fever," or "consumption" or "dropsy" (edema), or "scrofula" often called "King's Evil," a tubercular degeneration of the glands in the neck. Rather, we refer to those "minor ailments" so familiar to us all through the graphic advertising of over-the-counter preparations on television and in our daily press and periodicals.

Our forebears understood many of the old "natural remedies" for colds, simple fevers, headaches, sprains, bruises, burns, upset stomachs and "poor bowels." Many of them have been discredited. But many more have been "proved out" as sound medical practice. In short, over centuries, their effectiveness has been verified.

We find ourselves in the anomalous position of assuming that because of our great scientific and technological advances, we can safely believe in the efficacy of those "amazing new discoveries" in proprietary ("patent") medicines simply because great corporations with "fine sounding names" tell us we can—when in fact, many of the old home remedies were not only more sound (particularly in the treatment of self-limiting diseases), but more effective and cheaper as well.

If it is true that there was an element of "placebo effect" in them because we firmly *believed* they would help, it is no less true of today's over-the-counter drug products. In fact, there is much laboratory evidence to indicate that the mental "feel better factor" is much greater in today's remedies because of the constant barrage of subliminal conditioning through the printed media, radio and television.

Time and time again in our research, physicians say, "We are the most overmedicated, drug-oriented society the world has ever known." They say it with real concern. They direct much of their blame at the pharmaceutical corporations who have flooded the market with something on the order of a half million "patent medicines."

Many of these have proved dangerous. Under certain conditions, some of them turned out to be killers. It is a fact that, if abused, most of them have the potential to cause death. One of the great problems facing many of us today stems from our abuse—often unwittingly—of such commonly used drugs as aspirin.

A number of readers may be made "uncomfortable" by some material in *Pre-Medicated Murder?* Not all physicians agree with everything we have included here. Not all the scientists at the Food and Drug Administration in Washington, D.C., agree with all the precautions or with all the policies that are presently being proposed or implemented. Some of them are felt to be too conservative. However, faced with the alternative of commercially acceptable approval standards regarding test methods and the time periods over which tests should be conducted, and the very real tragedies confronting them in the case of thalidomide (an "ethical" drug) and the aerosol cold relief sprays (a "proprietary" drug), they were forced to err on the side of conservatism.

Every authority interviewed spoke candidly when we explained that the work was not to be another "expose" but rather an informally written *service book,* an espousal of common sense practices in self-medication (an economic and societal necessity) and professional medication.

After many months, when the great mass of material had been collected, evaluated and set down in manuscript form, we, being investigative reporters not scientists, decided to seek an overview opinion on the correctness and utility of the work from a friend whose distinguished reputation as a medical scientist is unquestioned.

We sought out Dr. Ralph W. Gerard, world reknowned physiologist and Dean Emeritus of the Medical School at the University of California, Irvine, with whom we shared a deep interest in the work of certain University support groups. We asked Dr. Gerard if he would read the manuscript and evaluate it for accuracy. He agreed despite a most active "retirement" in which his phenomenal knowledge and wise counsel was constantly being sought in medical circles here and abroad.

We write this acknowledgment with heavy hearts. Three days ago, on February 17, 1974, Ralph Gerard died in his seventy-third year after undergoing emergency surgery related to a long-standing coronary disorder. We take some comfort from the fact that we were able to discuss the manuscript with our friend at his home a few days earlier and say to him again, in person, how very grateful we are for his professional and personal reassurances.

Ralph Gerard understood that we, as investigative writers, made no claim to medical expertise; and yet he found that we have "...on every topic discussed, reached conclusions which are healthy and sound and on the side of the angels."

In our sadness, we manage a smile now as we recall that Ralph was not so certain that the title of the book and some of the chapter headings deserved "celestial blessings." "I am a pedant," he said (knowing we would properly protest), "and as such I am not uncommonly fond of the pun."

Then he added with a twinkle, "But you two were not really designing your book for so limited an audience as we scientists and professors, were you?"

Doctor Gerard credited us with "getting the feel and coloration of the subject matter in a truly professional sense," and added, "I read the manuscript with real pleasure and considerable instruction and am sure that the intelligent layman will find it a valuable guide to decisions in many critical areas of action in individual or public health matters."

We have no hope more sincere than that we have succeeded reasonably well in that objective. If we have, an enormous measure of credit must go to Ralph Gerard for his generous counsel and encouragement. His friends were legion and those who have benefited through his dedication and superior knowledge stand grateful, in double rank, around the world.

Having paid, in so far as we are able, this primary debt of gratitude, we wish also to express our deep appreciation to the scores of others who shared generously their specialized knowledge in the various areas covered herein. If there are any omissions, they are as inadvertent as they seem to be inevitable when thousands of miles are traveled, scores of persons interviewed and more thousands of notes taken.

Therefore, petitioning for understanding and forgiveness, we extend our sincere gratitude and thanks to:

E.L. Atkins, Attorney

M. Joe Brockman, D.D.S.

Cynthia Butler, Head of Public Services, Medical Library, UCI

Kenneth Carpenter, Attorney

Dr. Joseph D. Cooper, Professor of Political Sciences, Howard University and editor of "The Efficacy of Self-Medication"

Arthur H. Downing, M.D.

Dr. Alan Forbes, Acting Director, Bureau of Foods, FDA

Ralph W. Gerard, M.D., editor of "Food for Life"

Donald Heller, Assistant Vice President of Sunkist Growers

W. Ray Henderson, M.D.

Murray Hoffstein, M.D.

Dr. Ogden Johnson, Director, Bureau of Foods, FDA

Thaddeus Jones, M.D.

Charles Martin, M.D.

Jerry Meyer, Office of Legislative Services, FDA

Edward R. Nida, Press Officer, FDA

Mrs. Kate Oliver, Librarian, Communication Department of AMA

Mary Ritchey, University of California, Irvine's Medical Library

Edward Shanbrom, M.D.

Frederick Veitch, M.D.

John T. Waldon, Deputy Assistant Commissioner for Public Affairs, FDA

William J. Williams, Vice President, Irvine Company and Director of Sunkist Growers

Gary Yingling, Director, Bureau of Drugs, FDA

H. Mark Young, M.D.

and to the directors and staffs of:

Consumer Product Safety Commission

The Interdisciplinary Communication Program of the Smithsonian Institution

American Pharmaceutical Association Library

The Library of Congress

The Proprietary Association of America

The Laguna Beach Library

Pre-Medicated Murder?

1 Do-it-Yourself Destruction

Kipling claimed that prostitution is the oldest profession. Much later Alexander Woollcott would add to that the profession of acting and claim acidulously that both practices have been "ruined by amateurs."

With due deference to those two perceptive gentlemen, the preponderance of evidence places the practice of medicine as the oldest profession. And while some medical practitioners, in all ages, have been accused of prostitution and of posturing, there is no doubt whatever that most members of the bona fide oldest profession are the most dedicated and selfless professionals the world has known. Moreover, they are the only professionals who devote their lives to making their professions unnecessary.

"Truth in all its kinds," wrote Peter Latham, "is most difficult to win; and truth in medicine is the most difficult of all."

The search for truth in medicine that is carried on formally in the world's great laboratories and informally through the meditations, reflections, suppositions, suspicions, hopes and hunches of thousands of physicians in their private practices is one of the most thrilling explorations man will ever know.

The nature of the earth, the nature of a neighboring planet or of a distant galaxy, pales in importance beside the possibility that one day these dedicated scientists will discover all the essential secrets in the nature of man; for when they do, they will have freed man himself to unlock those other secrets of the Universe.

Some who read this are saying now, "Yes—but what about man's mind—his brain? What about the nature of that most mysterious human function?" The physicians and psychiatrists with whom we have talked are in complete accord on that answer. Once science has fathomed the *modus operandi* of the human brain—the relationship between the psyche and the soma—most of the riddles of the human condition will soon be solved. As one scientist put it, "We will then know which wrenches to use to repair which 'loose nuts.'"

As of now, the end of that search seems distant indeed. When we undertook our own quest into just *one* aspect of the human paradox, it soon became apparent that when turned loose in the neighborhood drugstore even the wisest of us become "card carrying nuts" who willingly risk permanent damage to our bodies and minds by self-prescribing and administering an incredible assortment of drugs, many of which can and will kill us.

Why do otherwise rational and conservative individuals take such chances with their most precious possessions, their lives and good health? Why do we insist upon diagnosing our own ailments rather than go immediately to a competent doctor? There are many answers, none of which can really be called sensible.

Older people who have the highest incidence of illness and disease, *and the lowest incomes,* medicate themselves through fear—fear of learning a dreaded truth, fear of excessive medical fees and associated charges far beyond their ability to pay, even with Medicare.

People in the lower income brackets and in the poverty groups confess to the same motives.

In the higher income groups, individuals who can afford the best medical care—the drivers, the achievers—do it to save time. "I'm too damned busy to be sick!" they boast. When the family physician hears this—usually too late—he will probably resort to the truism, "He took his fancy car to be serviced every two months, but I haven't seem *him* for five years!"

Ludicrous as it is when balanced against the facts, a number of persons resort to self-diagnosis and self-medication because of a mistrust of the medical profession. "More doc tors drive Cadillacs than anybody else!" "Doctors don't give a hoot in hell about the patient's body—just his pocket-book." Or, "Doctors won't examine your body until they've examined your bank account."

The currency given to these misrepresentations and downright lies is old indeed. Herodotus (484 to 425 B.C., or thereabout), from whom we learn most about ancient medical practices, observed this suspicion and skepticism when he wrote of the Babylonians whose physicians were among the most skilled in the ancient world.

"We now come," he wrote, "to the wisest of their customs. Having little use for physicians, they carry their sick into the marketplace. Then those who have been similarly afflicted come near and advise the victim about his disease and comfort him and tell him by what means they themselves have recovered from it or have seen others recover. None may pass by the sick man without speaking and asking what is his sickness."

How little human nature has changed with the passing centuries! How much this ancient Babylonian practice resembles the informal "organ recitals" that may be overheard wherever people gather—most especially in those places where older persons gather!

As centers of hearsay and medical heresy, the public squares of Babylonia have been replaced by our modern health food stores where, too often, inexpert and questionable scientific advice is dispensed freely to expedite the sale of thousands of costly foods and medicaments. They must as surely heal the manufacturer's financial ills as they fail to heal the physical ailments of the aging hopefuls who further comfort themselves by listening to the experiences of other self-deluded peers who are unable or unwilling to confess their own poor judgment. Over the years, the sight of these oldsters moved the male half of this collaboration to write a quatrain:

Elderly folks with fear in their eyes
Bending o'er tables of health food supplies,
Belying the maxim that ancient is wise
By gullibly gulping those labelous lies.

One cannot say that here and there—in Babylonia and elsewhere on down to modern times—bits of truth have not been revealed and passed along to comfort and perhaps to cure. But certainly the law of random chance is far less dependable than the possiblity that the disciplined science of medicine will come up with some definitive clues to the cause and cure of mankind's most serious ailments. True, some of medicine's great discoveries have been called "accidents." But they were the predictable accidents that always result from the orderly, in-depth pursuit of a goal undertaken by highly trained minds exploring the most likely avenues of investigation.

If there is one thing an investigator discovers early in his search for meaningful information in the medical field, it is the surfeit of statistics that are generally meaningless to the average person.

In *Pre-Medicated Murder?* we want to avoid as many "numbers" as possible and still make the central point—*that far too many* people are killing themselves by increments through the indiscriminate use of so-called ethical and over-the-counter drugs, or OTCs, as nonprescription remedies are known at the Food and Drug Administration where a significant amount of our research was done.

Nobody would come up with a "hard" figure indicating how many Americans patronize the local drugstore each week. The "guestimates" ranged from 120 million to 160 million.* If we use the median figure of 140 million we are told we will be conservative.

We do know that each year Americans spend $6 billion on prescription drugs.

Another $4 billion is spent on proprietary drugs and other health aids. (The word "proprietary" is the favorite euphemism for "patent medicines.")

One way or another, Americans pay for another $1.5 billion in drugs administered to them in private hospitals.

---

*In 1933 Arthur Kallet and F. J. Schlink of Consumers Research, Inc., found there were "One Hundred Million Guinea Pigs" in their book by that title.

As taxpayers, we buy another $.5 billion through federal, state, county and city purchases.

And indirectly, we pay another $.2 billion for drugs purchased by nursing homes and psychiatric clinics.

Our total ethical and proprietary drug bill comes to $12.2 billion. As high as that bill is, it's less than half the annual cost to industry of our indulgence in our *favorite* drug, alcohol! And each year, the bill is increasing because our population is increasing, because a higher percentage of our population lives into the retirement years and because scores of "new" remedies are launched with national TV, radio and printed media campaigns designed by the most skillfull "mind benders" on Madison avenue—the Mt. Olympus of the Advertising Gods but not necessarily their only abode.

Add to those reasons also, the fact that we are paying more dollars for the same old pills due to inflation. (What a boon it would be if someone would invent an ethical remedy for our nation's economic "flatulence"!)

The most obscure figure of all—and perhaps mercifully so—is the one showing how many Americans die needlessly each year because they have tried to diagnose and treat their own ailments. Intermittent and persistent headaches, burning stomach, sore throat, chronic head colds, apparent muscular pains that, too late, are identified as critical danger signals; referred pains from heart, kidney, liver, gall bladder, spleen and other disorders—all of these pains in their early manifestations quite probably can be made to subside temporarily by the use of aspirin and other analgesics that mask or suppress symptoms.

The temptation to indulge in self-diagnosis is made greater still by the knowledge that many "chest pains" are not coronary related discomforts but merely uncomfortable but otherwise harmless symptoms of a mild indigestion or an inflamation in one of the many muscles that sheath the skeleton close to the surface.

"I spent $300 on an examination by a heart specialist in La Jolla," said a friend of ours recently, "and it turned out that

I'm an air swallower. My diaphram was ballooning with gas and pressing against my heart and lungs. All I needed was a good burp! Three hundred dollars when an Alka Seltzer would have done the job!"

Because our friend is now in his forties, is overweight and works in a pressure business, we are afraid that he will ignore the next chest pains, assume (with some logic) that it's the same old "gas bubble" and discover too late that he ignored a bona fide warning that his heart was being overworked.

Most of us have found ourselves in such a predicament. For many reasons, we resist rushing off to the doctor every time we have a pain. But pains that cannot be directly and accurately accounted for—such as a stubbed toe, a twisted ankle, a stiff neck, a tennis elbow and especially internal pains—are nature's signals that something is wrong. If the pain is persistent, like the prolonged ringing of a phone or door bell by somebody urgently trying to get our attention, then it may be fatal not to answer the call.

Most physicians are as impatient with the stoic who bears his pains "heroically" as they are with the "crock" (hypochondriac) who calls at the onset of every twinge.

More than that, we are constantly being motivated by the advertising media to a high state of self-awareness. Velvety voiced pitchmen and women on TV and radio remind us that we ought to be glad that we are living in an enlightened time when we can talk about gassy stomachs, piles and constipation at dinner; and about headaches, backaches and sleeplessness at bedtime.

We have to "steel" ourselves against those commercials showing the miracles worked on once "worn out" middle-age women who throw their husbands around like an Apache dancer before dinner, simply because they've taken a shot of organic iron to replace the natural minerals lost during "the change." And everybody in the family from Father to Fido simply explode with vitality when they "drop" their daily doses of vitamins. And if you're drooping after a bad day at the Rat Race there is full-color proof positive on your TV screen that a good shot of the sponsor's elixir or his capsules, pills or drops will rejuvenate you instantly—if you'll just *believe*—and buy.

Given a choice between health and wealth, most rational people chose the first on the assumption that if one is in good health the other blessings can be obtained. So the makers and advertisers of some 200,000 proprietary medicines have a strong emotional hold on most of us—a very strong one indeed. If the thing man most fears is death, then it follows that he most prizes life. And his greatest blessing is good health and the freedom to enjoy life to the ultimate. Caught between fear and aspiration, and knowing that death is inevitable but that good health is not, man lives on the horns of a dilemma; and the horn that hooks the deepest is anxiety.

Elsewhere we will examine another fear that motivates a number of persons to try self-diagnosis and self-prescription of medication—lack of confidence in the physician. Economic status has nothing to do with this particular anxiety. It stems largely from the inability of the physician to isolate and identify a particularly difficult disorder. After weeks of tests and stacks of bills, even an affluent patient is prone to give up in disgust and experiment with medication that, in the past, has brought some relief. These last resort remedies are not always OTC proprietaries. Too often they are prescription drugs—pain killers, "uppers" or "downers" that have made the person more comfortable, peppier or more complacent. As a matter of fact, the scores of physicians we talked to in the months of research in many parts of the United States, cited this as one of the most dangerous drug abuses extant.

"How," you might ask, "can people get such medication when the prescriptions for such drugs are usually not refillable after the first or second time?"

Occasionally busy doctors will "write" for another round. Occasionally busy pharmacists will not double check the date of refill. A few who are willing to take a risk for more dollars will ignore the date. But most often the drugs will be obtained illicitly—particularly the amphetamines, Benzedrine, Dexedrine, Methedrine and STP; and the "downers," the barbiturates and tranquilizers that are sold by pushers in street traffic.

By far the greatest amount of perfectly good drugs in these categories can be purchased legally without prescriptions in many foreign countries frequented by thousands of tourists who stock up and sneak the medicine home through customs by transferring them to old prescription bottles.

In France, we were able to buy "uppers," "downers" and restricted nasal decongestants as well as antibiotics and steroids, just for the asking. It was the same in Spain and in Mexico. Usually the drugs were manufactured by American pharmaceutical companies with branches in the host countries.

Just as a "head", an addict, can always make a "buy" if he is in need of a "fix," so can ordinary law abiding American citizens find almost any drug they think they need simply by making a "connection"—one that, in foreign countries, is perfectly legal.

As Aesop said in the *Fable of the Frog and the Ox,* "Self-deceit may lead to self-destruction." Certainly there is no more dangerous self-deceit than to suppose that, with no training and no expert counsel, one can correctly diagnose and medicate or cure an ailment that can, for a time, baffle the most skilled physicians.

Drugs that can bring a patient comfort and a degree of peace of mind, when administered in controlled amounts by a competent physician, are a blessing. Often they will make an ailment endurable until a solution can be found. Often, in the case of terminal ailments for which science has not yet found a solution, they can bring merciful surcease from suffering until, at last, life ends.

But as surely as day turns into night, if we prescribe for ourselves and treat ourselves injudiciously, we are in danger of hastening our own ends—sometimes by years of precious and useful life. Every time we succumb to the temptation to "second guess the doctor," we take one more step toward self-destruction. As the late Joe E. Brown said in the classic tag line of the picture, *Some Like It Hot,* "Nobody's perfect." But certainly nobody argues that the trained physician is apt to be far less "imperfect" than the butcher, the baker or the candlestick maker and their wives and children who think they "know better."

None of the foregoing is intended to convey the impression that the drug industry is inherently a creator and purveyor of "evil potions." Far from it. If the research chemists who compound, test and release for sale proprietary medicines were not conscientious in their search for safe remedies, the legal departments of the drug firms would insist they be.

In the case of most proprietary medicines, the manufacturers are more than reasonably certain that if used as directed—*and not abused*—their remedies are safe. The drug industry and pharmaceutical firms—long time darlings of the stock market—have, as often, been the whipping boys of the consumer's advocates. Again, "Nobody's perfect." But neither are the manufacturers deliberately imperfect. Not any more. There was a time in the early history of American "patent medicines" when unscrupulous "Pill Pounders" deliberately loaded their products with dangerous narcotics and excessive quantities of alcohol to guarantee that even a patient on a "death bed" would note some improvement—until the "high" wore off. But that, apparently, has not happened since 1915 when the Harrison Act initiated the great clean up that the FDA continues to this day. In a subsequent chapter we, will report on the extremely important work now being done by the Food and Drug Administration in the review and reevaluation of *all* drugs.

Some idea of the *great* value of OTC drugs in general may be gained from repeating a statement made on May 25, 1971, by Senator Gaylor Nelson of Wisconsin, then Chairman of the Subcommittee on Monopoly, Senate Committee on Small Business, in his opening comments at a hearing on the

Effect of Promotion and Advertising of Over-the-Counter Drugs on Competition, Small Business and the Health and Welfare of the Public.

Self-medication is part of our health care system. For self-medication to work, however, it is essential for the public to have objective and adequate information about the products used for this purpose. If balanced and full disclosure is important for the doctor to be able to prescribe intelligently, such information is even more important for the average citizen to medicate himself.

At the present time, twenty-five categories of OTC drugs are being reevaluated by the scientists at the Food and Drug Administration laboratories. Later in the book, we will consider the drugs in these categories in an effort to assist in the task of raising public awareness of the critical need to know *what* proprietary drugs to use for *what* ailment, *when* to use them and *how* often. *And more important, what may happen to our health if we abuse them.*

2 *A is for Aspirin and other Analgesics and Antipyretics**

"Aspirin causes internal bleeding!" charges one set of researchers.

"Not if it is buffered to neutralize stomach acid!" counters another group.

"Get the aspirin out of Alka Seltzer," warns Ralph Nader's Health Research Group, "or take it off the market!"

"Nonsense!" cries Miles Laboratories. "Alka Seltzer is safe because the aspirin in it is converted to a different chemical entity when dissolved in water. Sodium acetylsalicylate will not cause gastric bleeding that has been associated with ordinary aspirin."

"If you use the *pure* aspirin, there are no significant side effects," claims another manufacturer.

"Hogwash!" disputes another manufacturer. "All aspirin made to USP standards is 'pure.' The difference in price does not make it purer or safer. You are just paying for fancier advertising!"

Enter the Federal Trade Commission with a handful of complaints issued against the makers of Anacin, Bufferin, Excedrin, Excedrin P.M., Bayer Aspirin, Bayer Childrens' Aspirin, Cope, Vanquish and Midol. Also named in the complaints were five of the advertising agencies who dream up the commercials for these products.

As of January 1974, no definitive decision had been made on the FTC allegations that the advertising is "misleading." It is still in the study stages. Neither has it been proved scien-

*Fever suppressors.

tifically that the pain killers involved ease nervous tension and help the people cope with the stress of every day living.*

And so it is clear that the most persistent headache in the medical profession, in the pharmaceutical industry and in the government agencies that regulates them is caused by our most commonly used headache remedy—$CH_3COOC_6H_4COOH$—acetylsalicylic acid—or just plain "aspirin" to those of us who swallow billions of the little white 5-grain pills each year, "for the relief of" headaches, stiff joints, fevers and ordinary nervous tension.**

Why the furore? Because for thousands of us, this "simple remedy" may create more trouble and discomfort as it relieves. The question to be answered is whether or not this is the result of inadequate research on the part of the manufacturers, unfounded claims and half truths disseminated by the advertising agencies or carelessness on the part of the users. A number of professional people, physicians, pharmacists and chemists feel it may well be a little of each.

Because aspirin under dozens of trade names is the most commonly used remedy in the land, it is also the most commonly abused. Taken in prolonged overdoses, it has been accused of causing death. Children have been reported to have died from ingesting candy flavored aspirin carelessly left within their reach. In extreme cases, it has been called (incorrectly) "addictive."

When combined with other drugs such as potassium bromide or scopolamine hydrobromide to form a sort of "super" over-the-counter remedy, it can become dangerous enough to move some physicians to say that it should be sold only on prescription.

Aspirin has been known to mask dangerous symptoms until a disease—often some form of cancer—has progressed beyond the point where even the most skillful medical attention can help. And because of its widespread use, by

*The National Heart and Lung Institute will study research findings that people who take aspirin daily are less likely to have heart attacks.
**The total amount is not measured in grains but in tons by the Dept. of Commerce.

doctors and laymen alike, many physicians call this "work-horse" analgesic and the various proprietary medicines that combine it with other drugs to relieve tension, upset stomach and headaches, rheumatic and arthritic pain and the pains associated with gout, *"the most useful and the most dangerous of the OTCs."*

The most common charge—the one that aspirin may cause internal bleeding—is the one around which appear the densest clouds of confusion. Some of the researchers even seem to contradict themselves in subsequent findings. Some have apparently changed their minds—both pro and con—depending upon additional research or experience with patients.

According to Dr. John C. Krantz, Jr., Professor Emeritus of Pharmacology, University of Maryland School of Medicine and Director of Pharmacologic Research, Maryland Psychiatric Research Center, "gastric irritation and gastrointestinal bleeding appear to be the most frequent untoward effects following the ingestion of aspirin."

Doctor Krantz points out that the medical literature of the past few decades is "replete with series of cases of irritation and gastrointestinal tract bleeding following aspirin ingestion."

He cites the research done by Drs. Alvarez and Summerskill as early as 1958, indicating a definite relationship between gastrointestinal bleeding owing to peptic ulcer and the ingestion of aspirin. Almost half of the 103 *consecutive cases* studied were associated with the use of aspirin.

Doctor Murray Hoffstein, Chief of the Outpatient Clinic of Mt. Sinai Hospital in New York City, told us of emergencies caused when coronary patients on anticoagulants took repeated doses of aspirin, or compounds containing aspirin. The gastrointestinal bleeding apparently induced in them by aspirin was accelerated by the blood thinner administered to ensure the free flow of blood through the heart and arteries. Despite the fact that a number of the coronary patients had been warned by their physicians not to take any other medication, they had taken aspirin because they "had always taken it." Some of the emergencies reached the hospital too late.

In the May 1973, issue of *Emergency Medicine,* under the title "Asthma Over the Counter," the relationship between aspirin and asthma is explored. When it exists, it is a very subtle relationship requiring the most skillful diagnosis.

Doctor John W. Yunginger, Mayo Clinic pediatrician, notes that, "untoward reactions to aspirin can take many, and sometimes fatal, forms. One of these—too often over-looked of late—is asthma."

The problem in pinning aspirin down as the principal culprit is compounded by the fact that a tendency toward such respiratory disorders may be inherited by children. Diagnosis is complicated by evidence that an attack may, in some cases, be related to analine dye–derived coloring agents such as hydrazine yellow found in many foods and drugs. A significant number of aspirin-sensitive children displayed a sensitivity to such dyes. (Many vitamins use these.)

Doctor Yunginger suggests that the only diagnostic recourse, if a physician wishes to isolate and identify the culprit, seems to be the systematic withdrawal of every suspicious agent *with special care taken to make certain that aspirin is on the list of suspects*—especially when asthma occurs concurrently with periods of emotional stress or fever, condtions that send most people running for the aspirin bottle.

One need only look at the "headache" section of any drug-store to see how many pharmaceutical firms offer aspirin for children in especially formulated, pleasantly flavored doses. Very few parents would deny that the habit of taking aspirin as a "cure-all" for common colds, fevers, aches and general malaise begins in childhood. Most adults have depended on it for decades because, for its primary uses, the vast majority have found it dependable.

Some clinicians claim that aspirin taken alone is nonallergenic. We believe it is as foolish to make that statement as it is to say that alcohol is harmless if used in moderation when it is a well-established fact that one moderate drink can "set off" a chronic alcoholic. A very close friend of the authors' wears a special wrist tag warning that he is violently allergic to acetylsalicylic acid. (His boss's wife wears one on her ankle warning that she is dangerously allergic to antitetanus agents.) The possibilities for unfavorable reactions to commonly used drugs seem as varied as the physical (and emotional?) make-up of the people who regularly use them.

"It may be bad for me, but I can't get along without aspirin," wails a housewife who suffers chronic headaches. "I couldn't tolerate the pain in my joints if I did not use aspirin," another agrees. "I couldn't get through the afternoon without these," says a high powered executive popping aspirin at the water cooler—after his usual three-martini lunch.

The point of the matter is simple; all of these people can—and thousands do—get along without their daily 30 grains of aspirin when it is established that they are risking gastrointestinal and other damage that can be far more serious than the relatively minor discomfort of headache, hangover and sore joints.

Though aspirin is often habitually used, it is not clinically addictive. If it becomes prudent to give it up—or to substitute a prescription analgesic—rather than risk more serious complications, it can be done with no particular somatogenic complications. If giving up aspirin becomes the "lesser of two evils," it can generally be accomplished with relative ease.

"I'd rather have a head full of 'rocks' than a belly full of blood" was the way one friend put it when a routine stool examination showed the large doses of aspirin he had been taking for migraine headaches were causing an alarming increase in gastrointestinal bleeding.

Later, when his physician put him on a trial course of another oral analgesic, mefenamic acid, his internal troubles appeared to worsen. When last we saw him, he was talking seriously about going to a clinic in Chicago that was reported to be having heartening success in the treatment of chronic headaches. "What other choice do I have?" he said. "Apparently I bleed to death internally if I take enough aspirin to help—or I get 'hooked' on codeine or Percodan—or the bottom drops out of me if I stay on mefenamic acid. Nobody knows what's causing these damned things. Meantime, I've got a living to make!"

Another friend, a retired engineer, with a serious cardiovascular condition that required a low sodium diet, nearly did himself in by taking an OTC preparation that relieved the pain in long inactive muscles but increased his sodium retention to the point where he had to be hospitalized. "I've been taking the stuff for thirty years," he said in an injured tone. "It's always been harmless for me."

Some years ago another friend, a nationally known dance director, began, in his early forties, to show a classic symptom of gout, an ailment that was once associated with "portly English gentlemen." The symptom, of course, was an acute pain in the big toe—a most inconvenient place for a dance director to develop a persistent discomfort.

"Why there?" he groaned. "Why not in my arm or in my 'tail'?" His physician diagnosed the ailment quickly and accurately and prescribed a diet low in food that produces high concentrations of uric acid in the blood and urine. To relieve the discomfort, the physician prescribed some rather heavy doses of aspirin; and during a particularly acute attack which involved some other joints, our friend was put on colchicine, a powerful alkaloid that has been used successfully for years in the treatment of gout.

After a few weeks on the low protein diet, during which alcoholic beverages were also banned, our friend began to show an improvement. "Funny thing about it, though," he said when he was back at work, "the aspirin didn't do very much for the pain."

In the light of new findings on the use of acetylsalicylic acid for the relief of early gout pain, our friend seems to have been making an inadvertent but important clinical observation. Although we found no great body of research to support the conclusion, several well qualified physicians are saying that while *colchicine, indomethacin* and *phenylbutazone* are generally effective in relieving an acute attack of gouty arthritis, aspirin has no value as a pain killer. More than that they state, it may cause more serious trouble.

During weeks of research in the Library of Congress and in the superior new medical library at the College of Medicine on the University of California's Irvine campus, we were amazed at the enormous number of publications, originating here and abroad, that exist to report the latest clinical findings. These publications relate to a near incomprehensible field of medical subjects.

Short of reading at least four hours each night, and attending three symposia a week, there seems no earthly way a physician could keep up with all the investigations, findings and innovations relevant to his general profession.

From time to time, professors of pharmacology sound the tocsin, making public assertions that doctors are lagging behind in their understanding and use of new medicines. Not long ago, one such doctor who is also the vice president of a worldwide pharmaceutical house charged that students are being inadequately trained in the clinical years, a condition he warned that could lead to a dangerous situation. If allowed to persist, the doctor cum drug executive said that the development of still more sophisticated drugs could constitute a hazard instead of a blessing.

A new kind of researcher is needed, he observed—one who is trained to inquire into the actions of new drugs on patients and record the findings for the use of physicians.

The doctor would also like to educate the public—to make people conscious of the work being done in the research laboratories of the great drug firms and to raise public awareness of "what it is missing" to the point where people will demand their physicians keep abreast of the newest treatments.

Man is depicted as the ultimate guinea pig. The clear inference is that new drugs should be tested on him—presumably after other precautionary experiments have been evaluated—for it is not possible, it is claimed, to pick up all the potentially dangerous side effects in animal tests because of "variations in the species." And in the end, when the drug is approved for use, the patient should be made to realize that it is impossible to rid all drugs—not even a simple old standby such as aspirin—of all side effects.

Acetylsalicylic acid, the principal component of aspirin, is synthesized today to guarantee a stable compound. Actually the acid was one of the very first to be synthesized in 1893 when a man named Dresser, studying broths and infusions of willow bark used in folk medicine for the relief of pain, discovered the "glop" contained a derivitive of salicylic acid. For over two centuries, Canadian Indians had used the bitter potion to reduce pain and fever. The recipe is presumed to have reached the American Colonies by way of a missionary. The foul tasting concoction was still in use on our ranch in rural Northern California a half century ago when the nearest drug store was a day's journey by horse and buggy.

From time to time, that venerable and compassionate "dean" of American internal medicine, Dr. Walter C. Alvarez, reminds us in his writings of the debt we owe to those ancient "natural vegetable remedies." As early as 1500 B.C., opium and castor oil were in general use in the eastern Mediterranean. The Spaniards found cocaine and quinine in South American forests. In 1776, Britain's Dr. William Withering began investigations of "fox glove" that led to the discovery of the drug we know today as digitalis—still a boon to sufferers from heart and kidney disorders. Ephederine, widely used for the relief of asthma and certain other respiratory ailments, was discovered by a Chinese physician in 1922. And not long ago, the lowly periwinkle, historically used as a medicine in some countries, was found to be a source of a drug called Vincristine, now helping to prolong the lives of children stricken with leukemia. Add to the list horehound, ginger, eucalyptus, brea and a thousand other "natural remedies" and one gets an inkling of how much even the earliest serious physicians had to "be up on" to ensure the most "modern" treatments for their patients.

Now, when we hear someone damn physicians for specializing, we are tempted to lead them to the 6-foot pile of new data related exclusively to the uses and effects of the lowly aspirin tablet!

When we began our research for this work early in 1973, it was a generally accepted fact that while the medical profession knew well what aspirin could *do,* it had little or no idea of *how* it did it.

Not long ago, the medical profession heard news that promises to turn into one of the most exciting and significant discoveries. In England, Dr. John R. Vane, of the Royal College of Surgeons, reported that he had convincing evidence that aspirin does its work of reducing pain and temperatures by blocking the production of chemical messengers called *prostaglandines.*

Although experimental work is said to be far from complete, Dr. Vane and his colleagues feel that these prostaglandines may be able to cause pain, fever and inflammation when they are released by tissues that have been subjected to stress or irritation.

Aspirin, they feel, has the property of stopping the production of prostaglandines. When this happens, the symptoms apparently are allayed. These curious "chemical messengers" were first discovered in the early 1940s; but during the world's preoccupation with war, the investigations into their character were slowed.

Now, with research accelerated, it is believed that they are present in almost all bodily cells where they may act as regulators. Because of their wide dispersion throughout the body, they seem to be active in dozens of physiological functions.

Researchers now believe that if they can learn how to control the behavior of prostaglandines, they may also learn, after centuries of frustration, how to control the functioning of human organs.

Doctor Vane believes that, in addition to other uses, controlled prostaglandines may be beneficial in the regulation of blood pressure and in the control of stomach ulcers and asthma.

Since the ingestion of aspirin is widely known to produce side effects such as abnormal gastrointestinal bleeding, Dr.

Vane, who is Professor of Experimental Pharmacology at the University of London, believes that stomach irritation may result because one of the functions of prostaglandines may be to inhibit the release of gastric juices. Since aspirin stops the production of prostaglandines which control the flow of acid, Dr. Vane suspects that the uncontrolled flow of gastric juices may cause irritation of the stomach lining. As one researcher said, "It's a bit of a three-cushion shot, but if it comes off it could win big for all of us."

Much closer to home, and perhaps closer to a practical solution, is another approach that, while not primarily an analgesic for the specific treatment of arthritic pain, it nonetheless promises as good or better a result.

According to Dr. Michael Reynolds, rheumatologist at the University of California, Irvine, College of Medicine, there is reason to be optimistic about the use of cytotoxic drugs in the treatment of rheumatoid arthritis. Cytotoxic (cell-poisoning) drugs are used in the treatment of some forms of cancer. They are used to arrest the development of "wild cells."

Doctor Reynolds admits that scientists do not yet know the manner in which the drugs work on the rheumatoid diseases, but he suspects it may be in much the same manner aspirin works. There is solid evidence that joint damage involves something called the "immune response" of the body. The immune response is the mechanism by which the body fights off invaders that cause cellular damage and disease.

While acknowledging that cytotoxic drugs can have very drastic effects when improperly administered, Dr. Reynolds believes that in the hands of an experienced physician the powerful drugs may relieve the most persistent symptoms of rheumatoid arthritis and perhaps even aid in avoiding permanent crippling. But apparently, as with the prostaglandines, the "jury is still out" where the cytotoxic drugs are concerned.

The hopes of those suffering from chronic headaches and arthritic pain continue to go up and down like a yoyo as each "hopeful" new discovery is fanfared and then soft-pedaled in the press. A possible remedy for arthritis was announced in the early 1960s and then "qualified" by a warning that while it seemed to be "the most promising analgesic discovered in years of research," it would not be ready for general use for some time—despite the fact that it had been known in paint and hardware stores for over fifty years!

The product is dimethylsulfoxide, more popularly known as DMSO. It is a commercial solvent made from wood pulp. Its curious painkilling capacity has been known since 1962.

Doctor Stanley W. Jacob and a research team at the University of Oregon Medical School discovered, by chance, that DMSO possesses a mysterious capability to suppress pain. Further research indicated that the solvent also possesses a capability of penetrating the skin to carry other agents deep into the tissues of the body.

Since the common hardware store grade of DMSO was hardly suitable for clinical research, Dr. Jacob and his team purified a quantity of the solvent to meet medical standards. The results seemed little short of miraculous. The news spread throughout the medical community, and soon several thousand doctors were busily engaged in testing the new drug.

The Food and Drug Administration soon began its inquiry in the interests of protecting the public from inadequately tested remedies. That was a decade ago. And still, despite reassuring clinical evidence that DMSO can work wonders with arthritis and that, in combination with other drugs, the "solvent" can bring relief if not a cure to other serious maladies, DMSO has still not been approved for general use.

Some observers claim to smell a plot. "It's as cheap as turpentine," said one disgusted doctor. "And that's the trouble. The big drug manufacturers don't seem interested. I suspect it is because they want to keep making other pain killers on which they have a better margin of profit."

Admittedly the charge is pure supposition. But it is understandable when many competent and cautious physicians, foremost among them Dr. Jacob, are satisfied that ten years of testing have turned up no significant side effects.

It must be apparent by now that contradictions and para-doxes are "a dime a dozen" in the medical field. One doctor charges that physicians do not keep up with the new drugs available to them; and another (the FDA seems to concur) charges that ten years of exhaustive testing is still not enough.

Perhaps those who err on the side of conservatism in ap-proving new remedies for general use are correct. Most ev-eryone remembers the horrors of thalidomide—a generation of babies doomed to live out their lives in tragically im-paired bodies. And who can count the suffering and secret guilt of the chemists, the physicians and the patients who believed it was safe? As urgent as the needs for new drugs to allay suffering is the importance of "being sure beyond all reasonable doubt."

Even a drug as old and generally dependable as aspirin was recently discovered to have still another side effect. New tests reported in the *Journal of the American Medical Association,* April 23, 1973, indicate that a number of com-monly used drugs can, under certain conditions, induce deafness. Aspirin was among them.

Of 1,597 patients participating in a carefully controlled test monitored by the Boston Collaborative Drug Surveil-lance Program, 17 developed aspirin-related drug deafness. The mean age of those tested was fifty-two years. Forty-eight percent of the patients were male. The figures reduce to only 11 per 1,000, a very small incidence. Moreover, deaf-ness attributed to salicylates are generally of short duration and are dose-dependent. The report states that "all patients in whom the outcome is known recovered their hearing."

The purpose in reporting the foregoing is not to level still another charge against aspirin but to show how much time and how much effort is needed to be certain "beyond all reasonable doubt" that a drug—even an OTC drug—is safe for consumption "when used as directed."

As it will hold true in the discussion of other drugs in sub-sequent chapters, the fundamental lesson to be absorbed is that of caution and restraint in the use of any medicine—but most particularly in the use of the common OTC drugs that we can pick off the shelves of our drug stores, supermarkets, motel desks and newsstands anywhere in the United States. They are old friends. We are easy with them because we think we can predict their behavior. And still, it is entirely possible that under certain conditions an "old friend" can be harboring a secret "grudge" and that one day everybody in the neighborhood will be shocked to learn that old friends are capable of "murder."

3 To Sleep: Perchance not to Wake up!

To sleep: perchance to dream: ay, there's the rub;
For in that sleep of death what dreams may come,
When we have shuffled off this mortal coil,
Must give us pause...

—*Hamlet,* Shakespeare

...and something else should give us pause too, and that is the strong likelihood that if we resort to drugs to induce sleep without strict adherence to a doctor's prescribed treatment, we are risking a very real chance of shuffling off "this mortal coil" without intending to:

During recent years, newspapers and magazines have been filled with the tragic stories of famous actresses and actors, columnists, writers, agents and scions of wealthy parents who have accidently killed themselves with over-doses of drugs intended to help them cope with tension by inducing sleep.

But if those tragic "names" are numbered by the score, the list of anonymous victims can be toted up by the thousands each year. Some hard figures were reported in the September 1972, issue of *California Medicine, The Western Journal of Medicine:* "In the year 1970 more than 7,000 patients were admitted to the Los Angeles County, University of Southern California Medical Center, because of serious drug abuse. A number of the cases were fatal. All told these drug abuse cases accounted for one-fifth of the admissions to the medical wards."

24

A check with county related medical facilities in New York and Illinois showed comparable admissions of drug abuse patients, percentage-wise, and doctors were all of the opinion that the conditions would worsen. Admittedly a great number of the cases involved the abuse of hypnotic drugs by young people who were "dropping pills and caps for kicks."

One physician made an educated guess: "If we are admitting eighteen to twenty 'D A' cases a day in this county facility, then it is safe to say that ten times that many are being treated by private doctors and in free clinics."

Eliminate for the time being those drug abuse patients who have taken a deliberate risk by ingesting (or "shooting") "uppers" and "downers" for the sheer hell of it and we are left with two classes of victims: (1) the person who drinks alcohol, then forgets that he or she has taken sleeping pills and takes a double dose and (2) the otherwise aware legitimate user who, too late, discovers the dangerous interaction of such sleep inducers as methapyrilene, salicylamide and scopolamine, common basic ingredients in the most popular OTC sleep aids.

If a person is on anticoagulants or anticholinergics, any of the barbiturates, steriod hormones, reseperine or tricyclic antidepressants may cause the most serious side effects including cardiac and respiratory arrest through drug interaction.

If that happens and no knowledgable assistance is immediately available, you are a murderer *and you are your own victim.* One physician told us:

> The great problem is that people who diagnose their own ailments and resort to the overuse of either prescription or OTC drugs or use a "friend's" prescription are usually not thinking straight. They are emotionally upset and physically debilitated or both. They are so involved in relieving their pain and anxieties that they seldom bother to read the ingredient label. And even if they do, it seldom occurs to them to check what other drugs they may be taking—particularly prescription drugs, or alcohol—that might interact. If your book accomplishes no other purpose than to start people thinking twice before they medicate themselves, you'll be doing the medical profession an enormous service.

We could have burdened the reader with pages of statistics and studies from a score of great medical schools here and in Britain and Australia and from the proceedings of such renowned medical centers as The Mayo Clinic and the UCLA Medical Center to name but two. It was necessary for us to read hundreds of papers to begin to understand the problem. At the proper place in this work, we will acknowledge our debt to them and to the professional men and women who explained and amplified pertinent information.

Instead, since this book is intended for *nonmedical profession* readers, we have chosen, wherever possible, to reduce the material to fundamental facts by way of sparing the reader the reams of supportive charts, graphs and reports that would require much translation from scientific terminology and jargon.

Because facts and figures become inseparable, particularly when one is trying to indicate the scope of a problem in terms of human suffering, we will occasionally succumb to the temptation and use figures. Unless otherwise stated, the figures will be approximate; since by the time any such fluid statistic is processed and printed, it is, perforce, out of date. Moreover, since the drug abuse problem is said to be worsening as our population grows and as more and more young people tend to experiment with illegal or illegally acquired drugs, including alcohol, the approximate figures presented herein will tend to be conservative. (That is journalese for saying the problem is probably worse than it appears to be.)

Eight hundred *million* drug prescriptions are written each year. That comes to four prescriptions for each man, woman and child in the land.

One hundred and eighty *million* of those prescriptions are written for drugs that affect the patient's mood and behavior—drugs that boost you "up" or bring you "down," to use a variation of street culture terminology.

The most common effect resulting from the prolonged use of such drugs is barbiturate dependency. The patient gets "hooked," in the parlance of the addict.

It is possible, by using related material from different parts of the country, to create an acceptable profile of the average patient who uses psychoactive drugs obtained by prescription or through illegal or unorthodox channels.

First, the incidence of dependency on analgesics and barbiturates is higher among patients with psychiatric problems than among medical and surgical patients who tend to discontinue drugs as their physical condition improves.

The incidence of dependency is higher among females than among males in most of the regional studies. A national study seems to reflect the same findings. Thirty-eight percent of U.S. women and twenty-three percent of U.S. men use prescribed psychoactive (mood changing) drugs. It should be pointed out, however, that this same study does not show a high incidence of abuse. Fewer than 10 percent of the patients studied revealed a dependence on nonnarcotic drugs.

While the figures in all the studies are consistent in showing that more women than men use psychoactive drugs, the studies of drug *abusers* seem to indicate that patients of both sexes, and a very broad age spread, are involved. Victims ranging from emotionally upset teenagers to people in their eighties are found among the inpatients being treated for the abuse of prescription drugs.

In cases involving older patients, drug abusage had continued for many years and the dependency, or the awareness of it, had sneaked up on them until they suddenly needed professional treatment for withdrawal.

It is important to remember that we are not talking about heads or addicts—drug culture street people. We are talking about statistically average people—the neighbors, the people we work with, our parents, our grandparents, and quite likely even ourselves.

We are talking about that nice old gentleman we meet at the supermarket and that attractive but harrassed young housewife who tools a station wagon filled with kids and dogs into a parking place near the drug store, and her ambitious young husband who is fighting his way up. We are talking about the boss who sits in those "pressure cooker" conferences and the salesman of domestic goods who is trying to compete with less expensive foreign merchandise. And we are often talking about doctors themselves—and very often about other people who work in the health care professions. As a matter of fact, in one very thorough Mayo Clinic study of 225 inpatients being treated for prescription drug abuse from July 1, 1966 to July 1, 1972, 31 percent were engaged in health care professions and 30 percent were homemakers.

Of particular interest in looking at an informal profile based on numerous published studies, and supported by conversations with a number of M.D.'s, were the "excuses" presented by the drug abusers whose excesses finally drove them to seek professional help.

Invariably these patients, regardless of age and sex, justified their use of psychoactive drugs on the grounds that the medication was needed to relieve pain, or insomnia, or anxiety and depression and, occasionally, nausea.

Most patients had used many different medications. The Mayo study showed more than sixty different drugs were abused. Sedatives and analgesics were the most commonly abused. The "symptoms" most often described by these "average" drug abusers were gastro-intestinal complaints, muscular and joint ailments, migraine headaches, sinus trouble, genito-urinary troubles, "slipped" discs, bad necks and a mixed bag of other complaints.

The great problem for the overworked physician is to sort out fact from deception through exhaustive physical examinations. Far too often, doctors tell us, these symptoms are merely rationalization—justifications for the use of psychoactive drugs—when, in truth, the patients were using and depending on them to relieve emotional stress.

In the majority of patients, psychiatric treatment revealed deep-seated emotional hangups. Without attempting to reduce a dozen studies to numbers, the picture looks like this:

A great many patients had undergone previous psychiatric treatment.

One out of four admitted to alcohol dependence, present or past.

Nearly all of those with jobs admitted that drug abuse interfered with their work.

Nearly all the patients confessed their abuse of OTC drugs. Usually they purchased analgesics and proprietary sleep inducers.

In all cases, dosage levels were dangerously excessive. An obvious fact.

Generally, the prescriptions resulting in overuse of a drug were obtained by the simultaneous use of more than one physician. One woman was being treated for the same ailment by four doctors; each of whom, unaware of the others, had prescribed the same or similar drugs at about the same time.

Patients who were abusing analgesics and stimulants tended to resort to illegal means of acquiring them. Theft and forgery were prevalent. As suggested earlier, the drugs were often obtained in large supply by patients who could travel to Mexico or to foreign countries where such medication is considered an OTC item.

Almost half of the patients had acquired college degrees.

Nearly half of the patients, when placed under psychiatric examination, admitted to unhappy relationships with family. Most of these were long standing relationships involving one or both parents. The complaints most often leveled against the "offending" parent were: "a domineering father," "an abusive father," "a selfish mother," "my parents were so strict we couldn't do anything," "I was taught that anything to do with the body was dirty, especially sex."

And finally, all but a small percentage of the patients were married. Two-thirds were unhappily married; about one out of four were remarried or presently involved in a divorce or separation.

After going over dozens of the studies available, many of which go back two decades and more, a vivid picture emerges of the characteristic drug abuser:

The patient is well educated;
Is married, or has been;
Claims an unstable family environment in the early years;

Has undergone some previous psychiatric treatment;
Disclaims emotional upsets as the primary cause of drug abuse;
Will resort to various kinds of deception to obtain drugs;
Will use a great number of similar drugs in an effort to find
  relief;
Admits that abuse interferes with job or career;
Is dependent upon a variety of OTC drugs, usually analgesics;
Habitually takes overdoses;
Is very often unhappily married.

The net profile shows a patient, predominantly female, whose difficulty began with emotional rather than physical imbalances but whose habitual abuse -of prescription and OTC drugs, usually stimulants and analgesics, has resulted in physical damage.

Time and time again, in the writings of physicians, and perhaps most often in the press, we are pulled one way and then the other by authorities with differing views on the use of barbiturates and other medicines prescribed to induce sleep. About once a year, the venerable Dr. Walter C. Alvarez will publish a column reassuring the reader that the judicious use of barbiturates—even over long periods of time—is beneficial to induce sleep; in our files, we have columns going back to 1963. And there can be no question that Dr. Alvarez's personal experience with barbiturates, which he says he himself began using during the great influenza epidemic of 1918, and the experience he has had with numberless patients are correct. This extraordinary physician and humanitarian's practice covers sixty years and gives us the longest continuous clinical experience compiled by a single physician.

Doctor Alvarez believes the rare cases of barbiturate abuse he observed involved "weak persons" who could not manage themselves. But members of a more recent generation of physicians point out that the spectrum of psychoactive drugs is infinitely broader now than it was even ten years ago. Moreover, the drugs themselves are more sophisticated. Add to this, they say, the increased economic and sociological pressures extant since the end of World War II and the advent of the atomic and jet ages—the condition Alvin Toffler calls *Fu-*

ture Shock in his best seller by that title—and you see a psychological environment that produces new demands, new dependencies and new abuses. More than that, these physicians point out, the proliferation of these drugs, and other drugs that might interact negatively with them, has increased the possibility that a physician may be "trapped" by a patient who is covertly using several drugs simultaneously.

In short, life and the drugs we use to cope with it are more complex today than they were even a decade ago. But despite the proliferation of drugs—*all drugs*—there is little, if any, evidence that any hypnotic drug is more capable of producing satisfactory physiological sleep than any other drug. Moreover, some of the newer ones have been proved dangerous.

Doctor Alvarez is correct in saying that the barbiturates are useful and in deploring the periodic "scare" stories in the press. "They (the stories) do more harm than good," he has warned repeatedly.

One of the results of these frequent scare articles in the daily press and in magazines was to set the pharmaceutical industry searching for nonbarbiturate sedatives. They didn't find one here in the United States. But in 1965, a new drug was imported from European drug manufacturers who had followed the drug since it was first synthesized in India ten years earlier. Its generic name is *methaqualone*.

Abuse reports were quick in coming from England, Germany, Japan, Norway, Australia and Argentina. Before long, scattered abuse reports began coming in from around the United States. Soon, they grew more numerous. One hundred and forty-six methaqualone overdose cases were studied at the Los Angeles County, USC Medical Center. The patients' ages ranged from 22 *months* to 80 years!

On February 11, 1973, the new drug made headlines when the death of David Whiting, business manager of actress Sarah Miles, was attributed to an overdose of methaqualone during the filming of *The Man Who Loved Cat Dancing* on location in Gila Bend, Arizona.

Los Angeles County District Attorney Joseph Busch called methaqualone "a potential death drug instead of a love potion" and urged the state legislature to pass strict controls on the sedative. The drug's abuse is now called "a silent epidemic."

"Love Drug" is the name the street pushers and users have given to methaqualone in the mistaken belief that it heightens both performance and the pleasure derived from sexual intercourse.

"Not true!" say the physicians *emphatically*. "Methaqualone is a *downer*. The best it can do is to relieve the anxiety that often accompanies sex. In that sense, it may superficially improve one's performance in that it may make one feel better about it—but not in the same sense that it makes sex *feel better*."

"Like alcohol," says an Associated Press report from Chicago, "the drug lowers inhibitions but also decreases the ability to act." The story quotes as its authority a group of San Francisco scientists writing in the June 11, 1973, issue of *JAMA*, the *Journal of the American Medical Association*.

Reports in *JAMA* and other related publications warn of the dangerously addictive potential of methaqualone and the possibility of fatalities due to abuse.

As with most new drugs, including the now older standbys, methaqualone has its place even though its abuse has resulted in clinically proved cases of physiological and psychological dependence. In Los Angeles County, four deaths were attributed to the abuse of methaqualone in the first six months of 1973. From July 1971, to June 1972, ten deaths were recorded by the coroner's office. On a population percentage basis, the figures were significantly higher in New York and in London. As with most drugs, legally and illegally obtained, the abuse rates are higher in high-density population areas. They are highest in the "core city" subareas.

For some reason not generally understood by authorities, methaqualone (a nonbarbiturate sedative), under its several trade names, is one of the most readily available commercial drugs on the street. Testimony during Senator Birch Bayh's subcommittee hearing on juvenile delinquency indicates a "significant diversion of the drug," which is another way of saying that a lot of it is stolen and gets into the street market through criminal channels.

Thieves managed to get 600,000 tablets of methaqualone from Parke-Davis Company by breaking into a warehouse in Detroit, Michigan. Police narcotic investigators estimate that the street price runs from $.50 to $1 each—a maximum potential for the criminals of $600,000 in a prime market.

Not long ago, a writer friend who prides himself on "working under pressure" came to visit us and produced a glass pot containing 200 tablets of methaqualone.

"Merry Christmas," he enthused. "I got a thousand of these on my last trip out of the country. Next time you get uptight about deadlines, drop a couple. They'll smooth you out right now!"

We declined in favor of another sedative we've used in *moderation* for many years—scotch and water.

The "secret methaqualone epidemic" has only recently begun to receive the publicity needed to instigate appropriate action. Far more common have been articles describing the use of "methaqualone maintenance" in the treatment of heroin and cocaine addicts.

There is much dispute about the efficacy of the treatment. Some users and ex-users tell us that methaqualone acts as a "booster" for the bad quality dope they shoot. Others tell us that it is simply a matter of switching from one drug to another—a case of which drug is available at a price and which dependency is preferred.

One manufacturer recognizes the possibility of *dependency* (let's not forget that the word is a euphemism for addiction!) in its professional advertising: "Physical dependence rarely reported. However, caution needed with addiction-prone patients."

Other manufacturers include similar warnings in advertisements directed at physicians. The ads also caution that delirium and coma, depressed blood pressure and convulsions may result from overdosing. Shock and respiratory arrest are also listed as possibilities. So is aplastic anemia. Patients on methaqualone are urged not to drive automobiles or operate dangerous machinery. Of course these warnings apply only to those patients who are apt to exceed the recommended dosages or those who acquire the drug without prescription and abuse it.

One street user was found to be taking up to ten 150-milligram tablets a day—in addition to the heroin he was "shooting." When he went to a clinic to detoxify, it took all the skill of the medical profession to keep the youngster alive.

Senator Bayh wants the manufacture of methaqualone slashed to one-tenth of its present production. In 1972, commercial drug firms in the United States produced 147 *million* methaqualone pills ranging in strength from 150 to 300 milligrams. The drug companies oppose the controls. They argue that it would "inconvenience" a large number of elderly people who need the medication; they would have to return to their physicians each time they needed a refill. "One wishes that the drug companies would display the same touching concern for our young people as they do for our elderly," remarked one physician who donates several hours each week at a free clinic. "If there weren't so many of these damned things around, the kids would not be able to get them. And there's no real problem about prescribing enough to take care of our legitimate older patients."

The inevitable conclusion must be a new sense of responsibility on the part of all concerned: the manufacturer who overproduces, the physician who overprescribes and the patient who overdoses. To expect any of this to change voluntarily is to confess a woeful lack of understanding of human nature.

The plain truth is clear—it is going to take control at all levels to halt the abuse of methaqualone and any other psychoactive drug. Obviously there are many more "weak" people around than the charitable Dr. Alvarez is willing to concede. It is equally obvious that they must be protected against their own "weaknesses." In our final chapter, we shall outline some of the possibilities that could bring about a realistic system of control.

4 "Let us Spray"—Aerosols —from Boudoir to Bathroom —They May Turn Your Home into a "Gas Chamber"

In July 1972, fourteen-year-old Tammy Braswell of Euless, Texas, a suburb of Fort Worth, found herself suffering from a summer cold. She sprayed a widely advertised aerosol "medicated vaporizer" on a tissue handkerchief as recommended by the manufacturer. Then, on her own, she placed the tissue inside a paper cone and inhaled. Within minutes Tammy was dead.

In January 1973, twelve-year-old Teresa Cummings of Richmond, Virginia, sprayed her pillow with the same preparation. Hours later her parents found her dead. The medical examiner's report listed "inhalation of decongestant spray" as the cause.

On April 12, 1973, five-year-old Marcia Overfield of Cleveland, Ohio, was put to bed with a light cold. She was given a handkerchief sprayed with the aerosol decongestant, as indicated on the can. A few hours later her parents found their child unconscious. The handkerchief was on the pillow beside her face. For five days, little Marcia lay in a coma. Then she died.

On July 3, 1973, the wire services carried a story that the Food and Drug Administration and the maker of the aerosol decongestant were taking the product off the market pending an official inquiry into the cause of little Marcia's death.

Five similar sprays were also removed from the market.

The product involved? Pertussin Medicated Vaporizer, a product familiar to millions. The manufacturer? Chesebrough-Ponds, Inc., a corporation formed by the merger of two of the country's most respected names.

Both the government agency and the manufacturer immediately took steps to recover or destroy as many as possible of the thirty million aerosol cans of the product sold since 1959.*

As of the time the product was withdrawn, the FDA said that of eighteen reported deaths linked to use of aerosol propelled materials, seventeen were the result of "misuse." Records go back only to 1968.

Attorneys involved in these tragic accidents disagree. They contend that in those cases were products were used according to recommended directions, no abuse was involved.

Meanwhile, the FDA has pulled twenty-two other aerosol products off the market for further study.

This "better late than never" process is reminiscent of the botulism deaths involving a gourmet brand of vichyssoise. It also recalls the scare involving one of the products of the Campbell Soup Company, later called unfounded.

One FDA spokesman was reported to have said that most of the early deaths were caused by kids seeking a kick. He suggested they were sniffing the aerosol decongestants in concentrations by placing their heads in plastic bags, much as glue sniffers do. That has not been proved in all cases.

Certainly it seems unlikely that young children suffering from colds would suddenly turn into "kick seekers."

Investigators may never be able to prove that there was not some degree of "overuse" of the aerosol decongestant in the sense that where the label recommended spraying the remedy onto a handkerchief for "two to three seconds" it was actually sprayed for "four or five seconds." Or that where the label recommended spraying an "average size

---

*On January 30, 1974, the F.D.A. also recalled two OTC aerosol asthma sprays believed to be potentially capable of delivering excessive doses of the active ingredient, ephinephrine.

room for six or eight seconds" the room was actually sprayed for ten seconds. But what about the reassuring statement on the label that one may "repeat as often as desired"?

E. L. Atkins, of Arlington, Texas, attorney for the Braswell family, asks a very pertinent question in discussing the possibility of "marginal abuse." "But should that kind of abuse kill a person? Was there any way for a fourteen-year-old girl to know that if she got a little too much of the stuff, it would kill her? I don't think so," he added.

Kenneth Carpenter, E. L. Atkins' law partner, added in a conference phone interview with the authors, "We contend that manufacturers are liable for injuries resulting from any foreseeable use of an inherently dangerous product with an inadequate warning, regardless of the intent of the user."

E. L. Atkins and Kenneth Carpenter are representing several of the "sudden death syndrome" cases, the pursuit of which through the courts may well result in a landmark decision fixing the limits of responsibility that should devolve upon the manufacturers of the drugs involved.

What are the suspect "killer" ingredients? Actually they are a very commonly used propellant and a solvent.

One of the principal ingredients, *1,1,1, trichloroethane,* is a chemical used as an industrial cleaner for fine machine parts.

The other, the propellant, is a *fluorocarbon.* The trade name for the most commonly used product made by E. I. du Pont de Nemours & Co. is *Freon.*

Over 2.5 billion cans of variou   roducts were sold using this or similar propellants during 1972. It is estimated that no household in the United States is without some variety of aerosol product.

"In cosmetics and medicine alone," observed one physician, "they cover everything from athlete's foot to dandruff."

The fluorocarbon propellants came into common usage during World War II, although experiments with antecedent products and variations had been conducted in the 1930s.

In the 1960s, some researchers were beginning to suspect that the propellant agent might play a part in what they called "the sudden death syndrome," even though Freon and related products were widely considered safe in "normal use." In fact, many doctors are now asking for a resolution of the industry's claim of harmlessness versus the fndings of investigators who have no stake in the outcome of such a study.

When used together—fluorocarbons as a propellant and trichloroethane as a solvent or agent to keep the propellant and the active ingredients properly mixed—there is now a growing suspicion that they might amplify each others effects.

It has been thought for some time that trichloroethane may be capable of causing respiratory arrest, apparently by decreasing the lung's capacity to supply oxygen to the body.

Fluorocarbons are known to change the heart's rate and its rhythm. If it is true that these two chemicals do interact to enhance each other's effects, then it is not difficult to see how "the normal use" of either, might form a lethal mixture when combined. Obviously, the same dose or application might very well affect users in the same age group in very different ways, depending upon the genetic inheritance and the physical condition of the user. But that possibility does not negate the basic reasoning behind Mr. Atkins' question.

"Was there any way for a 14-year-old girl to know that if she got a little too much of the stuff, it would kill her?"

Medicated vaporizers "for the relief of symptoms of the common cold" are not the only offenders. Bronchodilator aerosols commonly used by asthma sufferers are now a prime suspect in the mystery of the "sudden death syndrome." According to Drs. George J. Taylor, IV, and Willard S. Harris in a study released by the Department of Medicine, Section of Cardiology, University of Illinois Hospital, Chicago, epidemiological and clinical observations have related a significant number of these deaths to the overuse of these pressurized, aerosol-dispersed remedies.

"Lacking direct measurements, one can only speculate on the quantities of propellant that these patients absorb. Before death, some victims of asthma have exhausted two nebulizers in two hours. Others have been found clutching an empty aerosol nebulizer in their hands," the report states.

Nebulizers with wide mouthpieces are suspected of being particularly dangerous when a pressurized propellant is used to disperse the medication because the larger opening increases the amount of particles inhaled.

"Because the propellant gas is heavier than air," say the doctors in their report published in the *Journal of the American Medical Association,* October 5, 1970, "it may gravitate down the passages to the alveoli" (the air cells of the lung).

The medicated vaporizers are far from the only suspects. Aerosol sprays of various sorts are used for disinfecting bathrooms and kitchens, for eradicating or masking household odors, for cleaning ovens, for polishing furniture, for painting, for "fixing" drawings, for lacquering hair, for inhibiting body odors, for applying first aid remedies, for expelling shaving creams, colognes, after shave lotions and a score of other cosmetic uses.

Millions of tiny particles are propelled from the nozzles to hang suspended in the air, sometimes for up to an hour. These particles are often smaller than red blood cells. They are breathed into the lungs and often infiltrate other body tissues. The sprays are capable of damaging lungs, heart and other organs and, as we have seen, under certain conditions can cause sudden death.

Eye, Ear, Nose and Throat, a monthly professional magazine for ophthalmologists, cites a number of examples of women who habitually used underarm deodorant sprays and hair lacquer sprays who had to be hospitalized because of shortness of breath, general debility and chronic cough. Sometimes the damage is reversible. According to the *EENT* report compiled by Dr. Samuel J. Taub, in the case of a hair dresser who was exposed to the spray for long periods of time, the lung condition cleared up when she changed her profession and avoided the use of aerosol sprays.

Doctor Bertram Carnow, head of Occupational and Environmental Medicine at the University of Illinois Medical School, states that any aerosol should be considered a potential hazard. The particles expelled are so small that they can penetrate to the most remote reaches of the lungs where they are capable of forming scar tissue. There is also a danger that the minute particles can cause an allergy in some people.

We recall that some years ago an oil-based nasal remedy was taken off the market because of evidence that it could cause lipoid pneumonia. And still today, the market is literally flooded with oil-based aerosol sprays used for repelling insects and for killing house and garden pests.

A check of eye, ear, nose and throat physicians around the country confirms the dangers inherent in the use of any of these aerosol sprays. Three ophthalmologists practicing in New York City, Des Moines, Iowa, and Laguna Hills, California, reported treating a significant number of women patients who habitually used aerosol hair sprays. The complaints ranged from chemical burns on the eyes themselves to "blurred" vision. In the case of the latter, most of those complaints came from women who wore contact lenses and did not realize that they were hazing the lenses with particles of spray. After several applications, their vision was cut by as much as 20 percent. Fortunately, said the doctors, a little "window cleaning" took care of that problem! But the mist from phenol sprays used to disinfect rooms is another matter. The acid is capable of burning the delicate tissue of the eyes and causing irreversible damage.

Doctor Charles Martin, ophthalmologist at the Laguna Hills Medical Center in Southern California—a surgeon whose skill has won him international respect—acknowledges the danger inherent in the aerosols.

"I've treated several women patients who have inadvertently sprayed lacquer in their eyes while fixing their hair," he said. "But I'm happy to say that aside from a temporarily blocked tear duct or two, these particular patients sustained no organic damage."

While Dr. Martin does not minimize the inherent danger to the eye, he is far more concerned about the possible accidental misuse of the aerosol oven cleaners:

> These so-called conveniences usually contain powerful agents to dissolve grease such as lye and sodium hydroxide. They are

entirely capable of causing blindness. Like other potentially dangerous household aids such as the liquid drain cleaners, some now use safety caps that a child cannot easily open. Even so, I live in mortal dread that some day they'll bring me a child who has played with a can of that stuff and blasted himself in the face.

As it is now, our medical literature is filled with accounts of blindness caused by accidentally getting refrigerant gasses in the face while repairing compressors in freezers and air conditioners. Unless a corneal transplant is possible, blindness is almost certain to result.

Doctor Martin recalled that during his early days in medicine in Portland, Oregon, it took the persistent urging of a local physician to finally get the law passed that required the skull and crossbones and the word *poison* to be added to cans of lye commonly used in household chores.

"It helped where grownups were concerned," he observed, "but I doubt that it did—or still does—any good where a small child is involved."

We found few professional men around the country who were more aware of the inherent dangers in many of the OTCs and common household aids than Dr. Martin and his fellow ophthalmologists.

The point is that in this day of airborne pollutants and those expelled under pressure by commercial propellants, we are all in danger of sustaining serious eye injuries from foreign material.

Arthur H. Downing, M.D., M.S., F.A.C.S., one of the Midwest's most distinguished ophthalmologists and member of the Board of the American Medical Association feels very strongly abut the dangers of self-prescription and self-medication for eye injuries.

Says Dr. Downing, who practices in Des Moine, Iowa:

A patient may occasionally complicate or delay his recovery from an external eye infection by using eyedrops passed on to him by a well-meaning friend. "Here, use this, it cleared up my eyes in no time," is used as a rationale for treatment. May I say emphatically as an ophthalmologist, please don't put anything in your eyes unless it has been properly prescribed. Sometimes, a patient may call me on the phone and ask for something to use for sore eyes without coming in for an examination. This is always inadvisable and, at times, it may be disastrous. For instance, there are several conditions, such as conjunctivitis, which must be differentiated from a simple infection. The most important of these is a potentially very serious type of ulcer on the cornea due to the same virus which causes fever blisters. Another is acute iritis, which is an inflamation of the iris and related structures inside the eye. This is not an infection, but is related to rheumatoid arthritis. Fairly common are acute allergic reactions caused by irritants in the environment or by other medications. Patients put the most surprising things in their eyes. Other things which must be differentiated are corneal abrasions, small corneal foreign bodies, especially iron or steel and, rarely, acute glaucoma is first seen in a patient who thinks he has a simple infection.

In the foregoing, Dr. Downing explained why an ophalmologist is reluctant to prescribe without first examining a patient and why you should not use your friend's eyedrops. He further warns: "Your herpetic (fever blister) ulcer can be made much worse by the use of cortisone eyedrops prescribed for your friend's iritis, and the use of his atropine may do anything from inconveniencing you from pupillary dilation to precipitating acute glaucoma."

The doctor then goes on to caution us about the use of OTC eyedrops:

I am frequently asked what kind of eyedrop should be used to help keep the eye clean. The first and best answer to this, with some qualification, is "nothing." In a healthy eye, just enough tears are produced by the tear gland to keep the eye moist; just enough mucous is produced in the mucous membrane, called the conjunctiva, to keep it lubricated, and just enough oil is produced by the oil glands of the lid to form a top layer of oil to cover what is known as the "tear film" to prevent evaporation. *Irrigation of the healthy eye temporarily destroys the normal tear film and forces the various glands to expend much extra effort to form a new tear film.* (Authors' italics.) It is about as sensible to wash out a healthy eye daily or oftener as it is to advise a person with a healthy colon to take a daily enema.

Doctor Downing did concede, however, that this applied only to the healthy eye in an ideal environment and that our eyes, as well as the mucous membranes of the nose, throat and lungs, are irritated by pollutants which may cause excess tearing and mucous formation and thus disturb the tear film. He said that chlorine in pools acts in a similar irritative fashion and even clear water in pure lakes will wash away the tear film after swimming under water. The doctor then advised:

Medications to relieve this complaint are many and basically of two types: First, decongestants; and second, lubricants. Some of these require a prescription, but there are several available over-the-counter preparations. Most of the current decongestant eyedrops are based on a drug called naphazoline hydrochloride and are reasonably safe for ordinary use. These act by shrinking congested blood vessels for several hours and are free of most complications, except for rebound dilation of the contracted vessels after the effectiveness is past. This perhaps causes some persons to overuse such drugs. Better for prolonged use are the various lubricants. The best of these, obtainable without a prescription, are any of the various artificial tear preparations, which can be used repeatedly without harm. Also useful are the contact lens cushioning solutions (not wetting, cleaning or soaking solutions). I would like to discourage strongly the use of an eye cup with eye wash preparations unless the user is prepared to thoroughly sterilize it by boiling between uses.

What Dr. Downing had to say about problems related to eye glasses may well initiate another book; but for present purposes, we must continue with the subject of this particular chapter and discuss another distressing aspect of these OTC preparations.

It is difficult to know where to classify some of the products that employ the aerosol principle for application. One of the most troublesome but not necessarily the most dangerous offenders, according to gynecologists, is the feminine hygiene or personal deodorant that is sprayed on or around the vaginal area.

At least a dozen different conditions apparently resulting from the use of the sprays have been reported to the FDA. As listed in the FDA's compilation table, they include infections of various sorts; urinary urgency; open sores attended by bleeding and itching; burns, rashes and hives accompanied by swelling and itching; "choking fumes" and general pain and discomfort.

The *HEW News Letter* (73-28) cites 147 complaints registered with the FDA between 1969 and 1972. There is no way to estimate the number of users who suffered some degree of discomfort but did not bother to write. A Madison Avenue axiom claims that an advertising client may expect one thousand dissatisfied users for every one who writes in a product complaint. "It is absolutely certain," said an FDA official, "that the drug companies are getting complaints on products. And it is equally certain that they are not passing them along to us!"

On June 21, 1973, the U.S. Department of Health, Education and Welfare issued a news release stating that the Food and Drug Administration was, on that day, proposing a mandatory warning on all labels for feminine deodorant sprays.

To minimize any possible risk to users, the FDA would require the following language on each can:

CAUTION—For external use only. Spray at least 8 inches from the skin. Use sparingly and not more than once daily to avoid irritation. Do not apply to broken, irritated or itching skin. Persistent or unusual odor may indicate the presence of a condition for which a physician should be consulted. If a rash, irritation, unusual vaginal discharge, or discomfort develops, discontinue use immediately and consult physician.

The *News Letter* states that "the FDA knows of no *medicinal* or *hygienic* benefits derived from these sprays. Under the proposed regulation, the Agency will consider misbranded any feminine deodorant spray which uses the words 'hygiene,' 'hygienic' or similar words implying medical usefulness."

Products are usually tested as deodorants. This work is done in several "independent laboratories" whose findings are then held to be "free of prejudice" by the manufacturer seeking approval.

For any person interested in a detailed sniff-by-sniff rundown of just how this "scientific" evaluation is made on feminine spray deodorants, no more enlightening or amusing material will likely be found than Nora Ephron's piece in the March 1973, issue of *Esquire* magazine entitled "Dealing with the, uh, Problem."

Suffice it to say here that, unlike the tobacco companies who have mechanical smoking machines to determine the nicotine and tar content of their products, no such convenience has yet been devised for determining the relative deodorizing capability of feminine deodorant sprays whose primary use is to suppress or eradicate body odors related to the genital areas.

The scale of evaluation created by the laboratory "sniffologists" seems to be more arbitrary than scientific. Women who are paid to be test subjects in the laboratories are evaluated on a 1 to 10 odor scale. A test subject whose "SQ" (sniff quotient) is 5 is obviously a borderline case. The final determination is made after the test subject has been sniffed over a period of several days. Invariably, it seems, the tested product proves "more effective than soap and water." A debatable conclusion?

To return to the news release, it continued:

FDA acted on the basis of adverse reaction reports from consumers and physicians. The reports complain of itching, burning and blistering after use of feminine deodorant spray products. In some cases, urethritis and cystitis have been reported after the first irritation or rash.

Although FDA judges that the reported reactions are not sufficient to justify removal of these products from the market, they are considered sufficient to warrant the proposed mandatory label warnings.

FDA's proposal appears in today's *Federal register*. Sixty days will be allowed for industry and public comment. Comments should be addressed to Hearing Clerk, DHEW, Room 6-88, 5600 Fishers Lane, Rockville, Maryland 20852.

One New York doctor with a droll sense of humor who has treated a number of cases of vaginal irritation caused by feminine spray deodorants called our attention to what he called a "crotch duster" made especially for homosexuals of both persuasions.

"I haven't actually seen a can of it," he admitted, "but a patient said he had bought one for a gag over on Broadway." He said the ingredients were bad enough, but directions on the can ought to be banned as pornography. He added, "I wonder how long it will be before the manufacturers come up with a 'crotch duster' called *Fair Exchange? He* puts it on and they both get the benefit." (That led to some "creative thinking" that is better left to *Esquire!)*

The authors checked the best known feminine spray deodorants on the shelves as of September 15, 1973. In ten drug stores in New York City and in Los Angeles, we did not find a single product that listed the ingredients. As "cosmetics" they were not required to. We did find that most of them included a caution. When we asked one pharmacist about the cautions, he smiled wryly and said, "As far as I can tell most of the warnings on over-the-counter drugs are printed by the guys at county fairs who engrave the Lord's Prayer on the head of a pin. Legally, they're on there all right; but from a practical standpoint they don't do much good."

Even if the drug and cosmetic firms 'were concerned enough to make certain that the warnings and directions could be easily read, there is little hope that the average purchaser would pay much attention to the possible consequences of misuse. We are so familiar with these modern conveniences that we develop a sort of unconscious disdain for precautions, much as the average driver ignores the caution and speed limit signs on a parkway or freeway. (The accidents always happen to the "other person.")

Just what are the dangers of using these preparations? Mostly they are the ones already listed by FDA scientists who have cataloged them from written complaints.

But there is another danger. And it is germane to the basic premise of this work: if a woman finds she has a persistent odor emanating from the genital area and if she tries soap and water, and finally a feminine spray deodorant, and if the application helps to cover the odor but does not eliminate it, she should see her gynecologist promptly.

Some of these products may mask a vaginal-related odor for several days. But the product will do no more to cure the condition than will a Band-Aid put over a cut that won't heal. In short, the deodorant may simply hide an odor that could be the warning of a dangerous physical condition that requires immediate professional treatment. Just as some mouthwashes suppress or mask a chronic bad breath that may be the symptom of a serious gastrointestinal problem, so may a feminine spray deodorant mask a potentially fatal condition. Persistent warnings by nature are present for a purpose—as a preservation against serious physical malfunction.

Just how effective are these feminine spray deodorants? As previously reported, "the FDA knows of no medicinal or hygienic benefits derived from these sprays." The authors wanted to know why?

A young executive with one of the leading cosmetic manufacturers told us this: "We used to be able to put HCP (hexachlorophene) in our feminine spray deodorants. When that was not possible, we changed to another germicide. But the FDA charged that it caused liver dysfunctions so we had to get rid of that. Actually now our product is nothing but propellant and perfume. We put out one product that contains no perfume. The big mystery around here is just what the hell is in it—but the *propellant*? The chemists aren't talking, but so far as we can tell there is nothing in it." (The propellant itself is suspected of being an irritant in some cases.)

Under further questioning, the young executive told us that when these feminine deodorant sprays first came out they contained a variation of a "resin" that was used to kill surface germs that cause odors.

"Essentially," he said, "it was the same chemical that was sprinkled on the bodies of World War I casualties to keep them from stinking until burial details could get them underground."

He said the chemical was first used after the Battle of Verdun where two million French and German soldiers clashed; when it ended one million men had died.

During that protracted battle, Marshall Pétain coined the slogan, "They shall not pass!" Fifty years later, the FDA echoed it, in spirit at least, when their chemists ordered most germicides removed from the feminine spray deodorants. The "casualties" in the battle to secure the "home front" can only be guessed at!

Feminine hygiene deodorant sales amount to $70 million yearly. To make certain there is "nothing" in these products that can cause physiological harm, the FDA is seeking to take genital-oriented spray deodorants out of the cosmetic classification and put them under more stringent regulations that apply to drugs. This has already been done with antiperspirants.

Under the FDA's new categorial ingredient studies, these underarm deodorants are being thoroughly reviewed. The alleged abuse of these widely used products is said to have resulted in fatalities in the past.

It is apparent now that any substance applied or dispersed in or around the home by way of an aerosol container is coming under suspicion. Not all these products fall under the jurisdiction of the Food and Drug Administration.

On May 14, 1973, the Consumer Product Safety Commission (C.P.S.C.) was activated and given the responsibility by Congress of guarding the security of the American consumer in areas not supervised by the FDA.

On August 20, 1973, the Commission made national headlines by stopping the sale of aerosol-sprayed adhesives manufactured by the Minnesota Mining & Manufacturing (3-M) Company of St. Paul, Minnesota, and by the Borden Company of Columbus, Ohio. Between them, the two companies account for a dozen name brands of these convenient adhesives, among them *Scotch Spra Mount* and *Krylon Spray Adhesive*. The products—or some unidentified element in them—were thought to be responsible for genetic damage in infants.

The evidence seemed to lead directly to spray adhesives which, in some manner not fully understood, were suspected of causing abnormalities in the chromosome chain. The implied potential for causing birth defects was signifi ' cant enough that action could not await long-term confirmatory studies. There was sufficient information to move the Commission to warn the companies.

Acting with speed and cooperation seldom seen in such cases, both 3-M and Borden ordered their distributors and dealers to withdraw the aerosol spray adhesives from the market immediately. Executives from both companies, although confident of their products' safety, voluntarily withdrew similar industrial adhesives from the market until the alleged offending element in the products could be identified and neutralized or removed.

However, as of March 1, 1974, C.P.S.C. lifted the ban on the sale of aerosol adhesives. This decision was based on a review of many in-depth studies by a highly qualified panel of researchers. The contention that the spray adhesives should not be regarded as "banned hazardous substances" is consistent with the term as defined under the Federal Hazardous Substance Act.

Today there is a growing suspicion, also expressed at the FDA, that the broad spectrum of problems involving aerosols may actually lie with the propellants. If that proves to be true, one can only guess at the possible economic dislocations. Hundreds of aerosol spray products would be involved. Some magnitude of such a problem—and there is no substantial evidence yet that aerosols in themselves are the offenders—can be gained by counting the aerosol products presently being used in your own home and office.

We took an "aerosol census" of our own home the night before this was written. There were nine aerosol-propelled products in the bathrooms, six in the kitchen and house cleaning cabinets and fourteen cans of aerosol paint, spray adhesive, lacquer, varnish, metallic finish, undercoat, rust preventer, lubricant and house and garden insect exterminators in the garage! *Twenty-nine* "necessary" aerosol-applied products in what we often argue is "an average American home"! If it is ever proved that the propellant is the prime suspect, we imagine that between trips to the trash can we'll be doing many extra laps around our worry beads.

On the face of it, however, with aerosol sprays so prevalent in most homes, it seems remote indeed that, *if used with reasonable caution,* this modern convenience will turn out to be a poison gas. Such is the ingenuity of American industry that if there does appear to be widespread danger in the use of the present propellants, a new family of nontoxic ones will, in all probability, appear almost immediately.

From Watergate to waterworks, Americans now seem to be entering an era of reappraisal. Everything from pills to politics is under inquiry to the end that the abuses which normally proceed from the fallibility of human nature are corrected; until, and this is realism, not cynicism, it is time to do it again in the next generation.

In the meantime, use these "harmless-if-used-as-directed" products with *much more* reasonable caution!

5 Paying through the Nose

When the male half of this collaboration was a child on the family ranch in Northern California, his grandmother used to remind him of the dangers of abusing his nose during a cold.

To the tune of the old round song, *Row, Row, Row Your Boat,* she would sing with him this parody:

Blow, blow, blow your nose
Gently, without strain;
Otherwise you might find out
You've blown out half your brain!

Subsequently, when he forgot that graphic old melodic injunction, the boy, then grown up and pursuing a career in New York City, suffered through years of painful chronic sinusitis until medical science, new medication and a very perceptive doctor finally disposed of the worst of the problem with some very simple and sound "home treatment" involving isotonic saline nasal douchings.

There is no such thing as a nose that doesn't "run" occasionally. That is the normal state of the olfactory organ.

Americans spend nearly a half billion dollars each year for remedies to relieve or "cure" the common cold. It has been estimated that nearly every man, woman and child in the country has a cold or cold symptoms twice each year. That means an annual average of 400 million runny noses, hacking coughs and weeping eyes. And up to the present, there is no confirmed clinical cure for the common cold; although that glorious day seems somewhat closer as the result of some promising research being done at Harvard Hospital in Salisbury, England.

There, a protein substance called *interferon* produced in the white blood cells has been successfully tested on humans. The substance has been known since the mid 1950s; but early human tests were unsatisfactory. In the light of the most recent tests, it is now thought that they failed because the dosages were too moderate. Interferon is administered by nasal spray and it is thought to be effective in killing a broad spectrum of *viruses* that have been associated with respiratory disorders.

The problem, as of this writing, is the cost. Work is being done on synthesizing the substance so it can be mass produced in pharmaceutical laboratories. But at present, the cultures must be done in very small batches using human white blood cells.

The work, being done under the auspices of the British Medical Research Council, is said to be the most promising ever undertaken. Russian scientists have been working on the problem also. Using the same substance, they have achieved some success in combating the influenza virus—the area in which they are concentrating their efforts.

At present, the interferon cultures come from Finland where scientists painstakingly "grow" them in small, shallow receptacles that are not at all suited to the mass production techniques needed to bring the unit cost down.

In the meantime, while those of us who suffer from periodic common colds and related complications "earnestly pray" for the success of the British research team's experiments, we shall go on plunking down our half billion hard-earned dollars for remedies that do little or no good or, as one druggist put it, "remedies that sometimes do *more harm* than good."

Doctor Walter C. Alvarez, who has seen as many malfunctioning human machines as any living physician, says, "I know of no evidence to indicate that any particular food or vitamin is likely to prevent the coming of a cold or to cure it when it comes."

He goes on to observe that many treatments are used to block or cure colds but physicians wonder if many of them are effective. From our own investigations, it would seem that as many physicians are willing to state that they know of no remedy, OTC or prescription, that will cure a common cold

However, there are a number of preparations on the market that will ease the symptoms. As with all remedies that simply make us feel better or smell better or look better, the proprietary cold medicines may actually obscure the symptoms of a more dangerous ailment. They may also create a serious "side effect" in that their use may allow more dangerous viruses to get a foothold on the respiratory passages.

Before considering some of the common ingredients in these remedies and their effect on blood, tissue and mucous membrane, it might be well to understand the mechanics of a common cold and some of the cold-related ailments of a more serious nature that can and do result in an alarming number of fatalities each year.

Doctor W. Ray Henderson, a diplomat of the American Board of Otolaryngology who practices in South Laguna, California, calls the nasal mechanism "the most efficient air conditioning equipment ever devised." He says:

> A normally functioning nose performs instant miracles. Step out of a pleasantly warm room into thirty below zero air, as we often do in parts of the country; and within a split second, the nose "conditions" the super-cold air to precisely the correct temperature for the lungs.
>
> Or step from an air conditioned room in the desert into one hundred and ten degree heat and practically no humidity, and the nose cools and humidifies the outside air to precisely the correct temperature for optimum respiratory use.

Doctor Henderson admits that even a chronically inflamed nose is capable of doing part of the job:

> As a matter of fact, the nose is one of the "miracle organs" of the human body. It is infinitely complicated and we need to know much more about its functioning. We already know that some twenty viruses have been identified with the onset of the common cold and the complications that often accompany it.

And we know that germs normally present in the nose and throat can "latch on" and cause secondary infections when the thin sheath of mucous membrane is invaded and broken down by viruses.

Germs are often called the primary offenders; but they are not. It does little or no good to treat a virus-induced cold or otolaryngological infection with over-the-counter germicidal medication. The best they can do if they contain a bit of antibiotics is "zap" a few bugs. But the real invaders—the viruses—shrug off such medication and keep right on boring in.

Doctor Henderson agrees, however, that taken under doctor's prescription, antibiotics have an important place in combating germs when they are proved to be the cause of complications that may be related to an improperly treated common cold.

Given topically, orally or by injection, these so-called "miracle drugs" have saved countless lives by combating deadly infections in almost every part of the human body. But they won't cure a cold. To repeat, *they won't cure a cold because they are effective only against germs and it is now known that the primary cause of the common cold is one or more of the twenty viruses that have been identified as the real culprits.*

While we're discussing antibiotics, it should be pointed out that over-the-counter products containing small amounts of antibiotics account for less than 2 percent of the miracle drugs used by people seeking relief from colds. The balance of the antibiotics are prescribed by physicians for a variety of infections, including complications associated with the common cold.

Antibiotics vary in their ability to attack germs. There are broad spectrum drugs that work on the shotgun principle—they blast a number of germs. There are other, narrow spectrum antibiotics that are aimed at destroying specific germs. And there are areas in-between these extremes that can be used for multiple but not necessarily maximum complications.

The great danger in using antibiotics cannot be repeated too often: if used over a long period of time to treat a chronic ailment, germs can develop an immunity to it and the medicine becomes largely ineffective. (Also, some of the side effects—killing "friendly" bacteria in the intestines, for instance—can leave one more distressed than the original ailment.)

It continually strikes us as interesting how frequently the parts that combine to make the *sum of the whole* resemble the whole. It is entirely possible for a traveler who spends enough time in a foreign country to build up a resistance or an immunity to a "bug" that may, on his first few encounters with it, give him a horrible case of the "turistas." (More on the "global trots" later!)

So it is with germs that build up a resistance to the antibiotics and are left free to go on and do their "work." It can be readily seen then, that antibiotics are a mixed miracle that should be used with great restraint and only under the supervision of a physician who knows the *entire history of his patient.*

Healthy nasal passages are a complex miracle in themselves. Composed of pseudostratified columnar epithelium, they bear on their surface fields of microscopic cilia. Magnified they resemble a grain field photographed with infrared; except that normally the "grain" waves only in one direction—inward toward the back of the nose and throat. The cilia that comprise the "grain field" are bathed in a fairly dense fluid called mucous. This mucous is constantly being pumped inward and is drained down the back and sides of the throat. Carried in this fluid, which is completely changed once every hour and sometimes more often, are the bacteria, pollen and other foreign particles that constantly invade our noses with each breath.

In today's big cities, these hard working cilia and the protective mucous stream they pump are also expected to handle and neutralize a vast range of other foreign particles, especially those associated with smog and other airborne pollution.

(It is worth noting here that recent studies have shown that nearly 2 percent of the small children who live in central

cities suffer from near-lethal doses of poisonous lead, much of which has been absorbed into the bloodstream by the lungs after having been breathed in during their outdoor play.)

Normally these foreign substances that accumulate in the nose are swept along down the gullet and into the gastrointestinal system where they are rendered harmless. Because doctors understand this they are apt to give us a bad case of the "yuks" when they suggest that we should swallow the troublesome nasal mucous rather than risk blasting it into our sinuses by blowing hard to expel it. If indeed we ever knew, we forget that such a process is going on constantly and that we are largely unaware of it unless our nasal mechanism begins acting up.

Doctor Peter Lamy, of the University of Maryland School of Pharmacy, observes that the common cold must be one of the most "overtreated of all common diseases."

That is quite understandable. The cold involves one of the most vital bodily functions—the breathing mechanism. Interrupt that, even for a brief interval, and a thousand alarms ring throughout the body. So it is logical that when anything such as a cold inhibits the free flow of air through the nose and mouth to our lungs we build up an instant anxiety. We have an urge to do something, and quickly!

We resort to the handiest first aid we can find—"hawking and spitting," blowing our noses, coughing, reaching for the inhaler, the nose drops, the gargle or whatever.

No wonder we gladly (and hopefully) spend those half billion dollars each year for relief from the "common cold." Unconsciously our survival mechanism is warning us that one of our two most vital functions is being threatened. Never mind that the threat is really a minor one in most cases. We need air!

Why do we need air? Why are our nasal passages inflamed and plugged up? Because there's a war going on between our bodily protective mechanisms and some invading virus. And waiting in the mucosa are the ever-present bacteria, the germs, ready to follow the virus through any breach in the protective mucous shield.

As soon as the battle has been joined, some protective maneuvers are begun. Two conditions known as vasodilation and hyperemia set in. Translated, it means that the "tubes" through which the mucous flows are widened or "thickened" and there is a general congestion of blood in the infected area. White corpuscles are being mustered to combat the infection. The phenomenon is called "nasal congestion" and this is the condition that the proprietary drug firms deluge us with remedies "for the relief of...."

There is convincing evidence that a crystaline substance called "histamine," with a chemical formula as long as a "box car number," may be to blame for the phenomenon we know with varying degrees of accuracy as nasal congestion or stuffy nose or catarrh or rhinitis. That is why we are enjoined to take an *anti*histamine to relieve the troublesome symptoms. Antihistamines can reduce the natural swelling and give us some temporary relief by allowing us to breathe easily. But they can do some other things that are *not* desirable. They throw "road blocks" in the path of the defending white corpuscles and allow the invading viruses to get still better entrenched.

Once that is accomplished, the ever-present bacteria are free to do their work. And what they can do is give us "strep" throat, pneumonia, "staph" infections and, in extreme cases, open the door to tuberculosis and meningitis! Moreover, because physicians have such a complicated and often puzzling series of possibilities to deal with, the common cold may render the patient susceptible to a dozen other infections that can involve the throat, the ears and the eyes and all the interconnecting, infinitely complicated mechanisms that control them.

If the patient develops "viral pneumonia," recovery can be largely a matter of basic physical stamina and luck. Too often that stamina has been greatly reduced because a patient, instead of combating a cold by resting, continues operating at full speed. And if any of the other complications resulting from the original cold are virus-activated, the antibiotic "miracle drugs" would be useless against them.

It is clear then that the "common cold" can be an uncommonly dangerous ailment if reasonable treatment is deferred or abused. We can't be running off to the doctor every time we get a case of the sniffles. That is why most doctors agree that some self-medication is not only useful but necessary. But it must be equally clear that the type of medication we use must be carefully chosen. And clearest of all, if we are otherwise healthy, is the fact that we should let nature battle it out with the viruses and bacteria while we do minimal things to keep ourselves comfortable for the few days it usually takes for the infection and the symptoms to subside.

A number of OTC drugs are available and can be used—judiciously. As shown in Chapter 2, the most common analgesic is aspirin. It can and does help reduce the aches that frequently accompany the common cold. At the same time, though, it seems to give "aid and comfort to the enemy" by inhibiting the formation of *interferon*—the possible "true miracle cure" mentioned earlier—that is manufactured by the body to help defend the uninfected cells.

Nature devised the fever to accelerate the production of interferon in the body. By using aspirin to lower the temperature thereby making us more comfortable, many physicians now feel we are also lowering our defenses and laying ourselves open to still more serious infection.

The plain truth is that nature, in making us uncomfortable, is doing its most efficient best to win the war against invading viruses and bacteria in the shortest possible time. Our best chance to enjoy the victory is to keep our physical machines in optimum condition through proper cleanliness (especially the hands!), diet, ample fluid intake and plenty of rest—all basic things our doctors prescribe for us when we complain of a cold.

We have seen that antihistamines have no known therapeutic effect on viruses. But because they may help to dry out the engorged membranes, they sometimes offer temporary relief; which explains why, despite the fact that they have long since been discredited as cold "cures," these remedies still clog the druggist's shelf.

"Forget vitamin C," urge most physicians. Despite Nobel chemistry laureate, Dr. Linus Pauling's enthusiasm for ascorbic acid as an aid in preventing and curing the common cold, the consensus in the medical community is that the vitamin's effect is "marginal" if, indeed, any at all.

Doctor Pauling counsels massive doses daily. Many physicians counter that such self-medication may cause *cystinuria*, the precipitation of cystine crystals that form stones in the urinary tract. There is also a strong suspicion that the ingestion of massive doses of vitamin C (ascorbic acid) may make it difficult to run accurate tests for sugar in the urine, a critical test in the detection and treatment of diabetes.

Health food stores are filled with paperbacks extolling the virtues of vitamin C and nearly all the other known vitamins. In Chapter 11, *The Vitamaniacs,* we will try to bring to the reader a fair consensus of medical opinion about the use and the abuse of these vital substances without which life could not be sustained and with which, if abused, life might become difficult and unpleasant.

In the meantime, Nobel physicist Pauling, a host of naturopaths and nutritionists with various credentials, plus a goodly sprinkling of doctors, insist that vitamin C not only plays a critical role in the prevention of the common cold but also is useful in reducing its severity. To the majority of the medical profession, this is not yet a provable contention.

For a time, there was a great fuss in the proprietary medicine mart over something called *bioflavonoids.* Very early the organic chemicals that comprised the "miracle cure" for the common cold was given the designation vitamin P. Scatological humor indigenous to beer bars caused the name to be changed to bioflavonoids and sufferers from the common cold swallowed the pills by the millions and also industriously gnawed the white pulp lining of the orange in which bioflavonoids were said to exist.

Doctors are continually pointing to what they call the "placebo effect" of these so-called remedies. And bioflavonoids were given a staggering amount of undeserved credit simply because patients were "convinced" that the remedy was helping them.

Metaphysicians call this placebo effect "mind over matter." If you *think* you feel better you *do* feel better. Undoubtedly, after the third day, some improvement was noticed and was attributed to the new "miracle remedy." The point is, doctors say, the patient would have felt better if he had taken gumdrops instead because the common cold was beginning to run its course. It is a self-limited disease.

Five years ago, the National Research Council completed an exhaustive series of tests on bioflavonoids and determined that they were totally ineffective "for use in man for any condition." Since that finding was released and widely published, fewer and fewer bioflavonoid preparations are on drug store shelves.

A topical preparation is one that can be applied directly to the infected area. Nose drops fall into this category. As we have seen previously a very complicated "mechanical" process continually goes on in our noses. This process is speeded up when the common cold strikes. We have seen also that at present there exists no proprietary or prescription preventive or cure for the common cold. And we have seen too that most doctors advise letting nature do the combating—unless there is evidence of complications—or a sound medical suspicion that complications may set in.

Any remedy, topical or otherwise, that inhibits or restricts the natural defenses against the cold virus, and any hitch-hiking germs, is, perforce, useless—unless it is used sparingly for temporary relief of symptoms only. We've seen that antihistamines are often used for their drying effect.

Nose drops are called *sympathomimetic* vasoconstrictors.* The most widely used ones are OTC remedies obtainable in any drugstore. They exert a constricting or shrinking action on the mucous membranes in the nasal passage and, in effect, open them up.

They should never be used more than three or four times in any twenty-four-hour period. If they are abused, a num-

*Simulating or "miming" normal sympathetic nervous reaction in various parts of the body.

ber of things ranging from troublesome to serious may result.

Moreover, the more frequently they are used, the less effective they are. In addition to shrinking the membranes in the nose, they may also paralyze the cilia, the microscopic "pumps" that keep the infected mucous moving toward the back of the throat so it can enter the gastrointestinal tract and be disposed of naturally.

One of the old-time remedies still employed by many to help unstuff the nose is to apply one of the aromatic petroleum jelly products by fingertip or by Q-tip.

For a brief moment the eucalyptus or menthol or camphor or benzoin seems to give us relief. But in a very short while, the petroleum jelly is melted by the body heat, reduced to an oil and spread through the nasal passages.

There is clear clinical evidence that this is a very poor topical treatment. Tests have shown that oils, particularly the petroleum derivatives (mineral oils), slow down and often stop the cilary action and build a barrier between the infected membranes and any useful medication that oily drops may contain. Also, the oil may reach the back of the throat and go down into the stomach where the aromatics in it may cause other difficulties such as upset stomach. A peptic ulcer can be reactivated or further aggravated if the medication reaches it.

There are a number of vasoconstrictors available on prescription. They are infinitely preferable to the proprietary products for two reasons: the doctor will know of the possibility of dangerous side effects and will make an evaluation and choose the best one for the individual patient, and he will limit the amount of the medication that can be obtained.

Not generally recognized is the ability of most of the OTC and prescription preparations to become habit forming in the sense that if used for a chronic condition the user may come to depend upon them for relief and, in the end, defeat their effect by abusing them.

Among the side effects experienced by patients who use OTC nasal sprays and drops are cardiac palpitation—dangerous if a coronary condition exists—a general feeling of jumpiness, possible retention of urine and hives.

One of the greatest arguments against the use of proprietary nasal decongestants involves our inability to distinguish between what is really simply a common cold and what is an allergy that acts like a cold. And therein lies another good reason for making certain by consulting your physician. It is entirely possible that he or she may tell you to run down to the drugstore and get a small bottle of decongestant rather than prescribe one of the far stronger ethical preparations. But in that case, the physician will probably also caution you against overuse.

If a patient is being treated for diabetes or urinary disorders, the physician will, in nearly every instance, prescribe the most conservative treatment—nasal douches or "washings" with a mild solution of warm salt water—and patience.

Particularly dangerous to a diabetic are the oral vasoconstrictors. These pathomimetic chemicals, working through the bloodstream, can be effective in opening up the nasal passages and providing some relief. And it s generally believed that while they are less efficient than the topically applied ones, they are also less apt to be harmful to the membranes in the nasal passages if abused.

But it has been shown that these sympathomimetic medicines may also interact to reduce the effect of insulin in diabetic patients and thereby raise blood sugar to potentially lethal levels.

A patient with diabetes or a suspected tendency toward this all too common disease must be extremely cautious about the use of such drugs and must *never* "borrow a friend's prescription." As a matter of fact, it cannot be said too often that using another person's prescription medicine—even that of a close member of the family who may appear to have the "same thing"—is extremely foolish.

A generation ago in the authors' own family, two serious illnesses occurred because it was too much trouble to drive into town to see the doctor. One involved digitalis for a heart ailment and the other, a synthetic thyroid remedy.

These were intelligent persons who simply assumed, quite logically, that their symptoms were those of ailments that seemed to run in the family. Mercifully, medical help was summoned in time. In both cases, extensive physical examinations showed that neither person had any need at all to worry about heart or thyroid troubles. In both cases the gastrointestinal systems were "out of whack," and not seriously either. A few less fried foods in one case and a little less food overall in the other "cured" both persons.

Incidentally, in this same home, whenever any member of the family had the symptoms of a head cold, the kettle went on the stove and soon the ailing patient had his or her head over a basin of steaming water. With a towel over the head to trap the steam, the victim would inhale slowly and regularly for five or ten minutes with the hot water being replaced from time to time.

Today it is far easier to treat the symptoms of a head cold or a stuffy chest with steam. There are two basic types of vaporizers on the market: the hot steam vaporizer and the so-called "cool mist" vaporizers.

While it is not the purpose of this work to become a "home treatment encyclopedia," it is worth saying that both types are equally effective and may be used to hasten the body's natural "bug fighting" processes.

Pharmacists and physicians contacted were unanimous in the opinion that the steam does the trick and that the addition of aromatics has no therapeutic value whatever. "Put it in if you think it makes you feel better, but you're really better off without it," said one senior pharmacist with a national drug retail chain. "But don't put in too much. The steam is the important thing. The heat and humidification help the body do its job."

The steam has no therapeutic value either, it is said. In the 1973 edition of *The Handbook For Non-Prescription Drugs*, Dr. Peter Lamy writes:

Camphor, menthol and other volative ingredients when applied locally will affect cilary movement adversely; but vapors of these substances have no effect on the cilia. Thus, it would seem that moisture, when applied at the appearance of the first symptoms, has no curative action but can act as a prophylactic, permitting the cilia, immobilized by dryness, to return to their normal action.

In short, Dr. Lamy is confirming the opinion that steam's primary function is to aid nature's normal process of combating the infection. This would seem to confirm the opinion of a number of physicians who concede that, if given a chance, "Nature is its own best doctor."

That homily is deceptively simple however; and it presumes some understanding on the part of the patient that nature should be allowed to function as its own best doctor only after the doctor identifies and confirms the seriousness of the illness and possibly prescribes medication to assist nature in its battle. We have visited health food stores many times and heard clerks, whose sole qualifications were professional-looking smocks and a sympathetic expression, "prescribe" natural remedies after listening to some ailing elder's description of symptoms.

Some doctors admit that a good part of the practice of medicine involves the treatment of symptoms. But a symptom cannot be evaluated at a health food counter. They are often complex, deceptive and *apparently* unrelated to the real cause. It takes a skilled physician—sometimes a team of them using modern laboratory techniques—to make a proper diagnosis.

Once again, even with the so-called "common cold," it is dangerous to undertake self-medication. The cold might be an *uncommon cold* involving several viruses and a mixed bag of indigenous germs that rush into the breach in nature's defenses.

It would take a book, literally, to do justice to the exciting research being done on various aspects of the common cold and how they may be prevented and cured.

One of the principal objectives of research teams is a dependable method of differentiating between cold infections caused by viruses and those caused by bacteria.

It is important for the physician to know the primary cause. If the infection is caused by bacteria, antibiotics can be employed effectively.

But if the infection is viral, as it most often seems to be, antibiotics are useless. Moreover, as we have seen, they tend to weaken the body's natural defenses against viruses.

One of the body's primary defenses against infections are lymphocytes—white blood cells. These "white knights" of the body's immune system are divided into two classes. One class called B cells specializes in fighting bacterial infections. A second class called T cells singles out the viruses for destruction.

It seems certain now that antibiotics taken unnecessarily can inhibit the usefulness of the T cells and reduce their efficiency in fighting viral infections.

One of the reasons doctors are alarmed about the tendency to overuse the antibiotics, or to use them without certain knowledge of the cause of the infection, is a growing suspicion that some forms of cancer may be caused by viruses.

If this proves to be true, and in tests on animals there is evidence that it is, we are on the verge of a major breakthrough in the war against man's most dreadful killer.

It follows then that anything that may unnecessarily inhibit the activity of the T cells in combating viral infection may actually be inhibiting the body's immune system in its fight against a cancer-causing virus as well.

Doctor Joseph Wybran, a University of California research scientist working with a team of immunologists in San Francisco, examined a number of patients with newly diagnosed cases of cancer.

In two hundred cases, he found that over 60 percent had a decreased number of T cells which would seem to indicate that an inhibited immunity mechanism may have been the reason they contracted cancer.

As of mid-summer, 1973, twelve of the patients with a low number of active T cells died. In the same study period, approximately one and a half years, only one of the patients with a high number of the lymphocytes died.

Thirty of the observed patients who had been "cured" for more than a year showed a normal count of active T cells. Doctor Wybran has reached the conclusion that T cells are extremely important in killing tumor cells. "Without them," he said, "it is apparent that the tumors will grow."

What a tragic mistake it would be to use medication to cure a cold only to find out that, indirectly, it allowed a cancer-causing virus to develop. Surely there is enough evidence now to warrant extreme caution in the self-diagnosis and medication of the common cold. To do otherwise is to risk burning the house down to get rid of the roaches!

Like that wonderful old spiritual that tells us that "the knee bone is connected to the thigh bone," the nose is connected to the throat.

Any person suffering from a cold will confirm the connection between a sore throat and a runny nose because a feeling of dryness and sore throat are usually early signs that the "bug" has struck again.

If one goes to any large drugstore or supermarket, it is possible to buy five gallons of gargle, antiseptic or mouthwash without once repeating a brand name. But if you buy them to cure a sore throat, the truth is they don't work. Despite some of the most ingenious "weasel wording" in the pharmaceutical industry, these "for the relief of" remedies are seldom more effective than gargling with warm salt water or, for that matter, water alone.

Preparations containing alcohol have some germicidal value in that alcohol, in concentrations above 60 percent, will kill some of the bacteria normally present in the mouth and throat within a few seconds. But none of the preparations are known to kill viruses, according to researchers, and none of them will kill all the germs present in the throat and in the nasopharynx, that hard-to-get-at area "up in back of the throat."

As a matter of practical fact, gargling is a very inefficient way to treat the throat. Its cleaning ability is simply not related to the amount of noise it makes. On the contrary, the strong "burbling" tends to keep the medication away from the inflamed tissues. It is far better to gargle gently and bathe the tissues in salt water or whatever one's choice may be.

Most of the commercial mouthwashes and gargles do have one verifiable effect, they can and often do help get rid of that "dark brown morning taste" and the bad breath that often accompanies the decaying of food particles left in the mouth after eating. And the preparations containing alcohol or phenol or other known antiseptics will kill some of the "staph" and "strep" germs normally present in the mouth and throat. But most of the germs are hidden in deep folds in the membrane lining of the nose and throat and are not reached at all.

A number of physicians recommend a more efficient irrigation technique. It involves getting an inexpensive douche or enema bag from the drugstore and keeping it especially for the treatment of sore throat.

By using the small "anal tip," one can produce a reasonably strong jet of warm salt water that can be directed against the hard to reach tissues behind the uvula (the little "dingus" that hangs down in our throats) and in the far back areas.

The jet action dislodges far more offending bacteria than simple gargling and it also keeps a constant stream of soothing warm water and medication, if one is included, bathing the inflamed tissues.

Doctor Murray Grossan of the Westchester-Sepulveda Medical Center in Los Angeles reports a better idea. Doctor Grossan and a number of his colleagues use one of the intermittent jet action dental cleaners such as the Water Pic to propel the soothing fluids onto the infected areas.

The pulsing action of the warm water—up to 1,200 per minute with a peak PSI (pounds per square inch) of 80—drove far more bacteria out of the infected area than the ordinary method of gargling. As a matter of fact, in his article in the August 1972, issue of *Eye, Ear, Nose and Throat*, Dr. Grossan states that he constantly urges his patients not to gargle. "I regularly see several patients weekly who started out with a

simple cold and proceeded to gargle vigorously and then developed hoarseness. Had they refrained from gargling, they
would not have developed this traumatic type of hoarseness."

In checking with colleagues whose patients use the pul-
sating irrigation devices on their inflamed throats, Dr. Grossan found no cases where this mode of treatment made the
conditions worse. On the contrary, he reports that the majority of patients said they had obtained quick relief.

Even so, treatment of the throat requires the same precautions that other topical treatment for the common cold requires, and for all the same reasons. If you diagnose
yourself, and you are wrong, you run the risk of parlaying
that troublesome cold into far more serious illnesses.

6 *In Search of the "Perfect" Bowel Movement*

Doctor Jean Mayer, Professor of Nutrition at Harvard University, is reported to have observed, "There's only one good thing I can think of to say about the new freedom and permissiveness of today's movies, and that is that at long last our film heroes and heroines are allowed to admit openly that people occasionally have to go to the bathroom."

As great as our present preoccupation with other portions of the anatomy, certainly the sharpest, most persistent focus has always been on the gastrointestinal mechanism.

If we go back through old publications that advertised patent medicines, a fascinating excursion, we find at least three out of four of the miracle remedies dealt with the stomach and the intestines. In the days before the Food and Drug Administration began to police the advertising excesses of these doctors, bogus and otherwise, who compounded their felonies in the name of patent medicine, it was possible to buy one remedy that would cure everything from flatulence to flat feet. There were purgatives recommended for the "cure of diarrhea." Pills promised to cure cancer of the stomach and intestines, but the maker would not be responsible for cancer that might break out in new areas—"unless the patient takes at least *three* bottles of our medicine."

Claims are more moderate now. But proprietary remedies are more numerous. And the advertising media is more efficient. Who can resist the implied promises in those color TV commercials showing attractive middle age couples effecting dramatic personality changes after taking a tablet or a tablespoon of some remedy that "assists nature in her normal function"? Hand in hand, they walk along the fairway of a beautiful golf course, shooting sub-par golf and feeling well above par because they are "normal again."

Most of the commercials are directed at the older viewers, since it is presumed that people in their middle years suffer most from "irregularity." That is not entirely true. Closer to the truth is the contention that most younger people who work in pressure positions are either laying the groundwork for bowel trouble later or are already well into disorders which they simply ignore as long as they can. In that case, by the time they are able to walk hand in hand along the fairways, they probably are in a fair way to having chronic constipation.

Fortunately for most people so afflicted, nature will take care of the problem with a little cooperation from the sufferer—if the condition has not persisted so long that physical damage has been done.

It is easy for a busy executive or a hyperactive housewife to slip into bad habits that can lead to present discomforts and future trouble.

"I'm sick and tired of lugging around 26 feet of misery," moaned the advertising director of a large automobile maker in Detroit. "This damned gut of mine never gives me a minute's peace and it *always* kicks up just when pressure around here is heaviest!"

Certainly if the "hip bone is connected to the thigh bone" then the thought process is connected to the peristaltic process. If this harassed man had been able to think as objectively about his physical machine as he could about the 1974 models about to be introduced, he would have seen the obvious relationship between emotional stress and his obstreperous gut.

In his New York advertising agency days, the male half of this collaboration worked with these hard driving executives. Indeed he was one himself, until he opted out of the rat race. There is no question that nine out of ten of these men complained of intestinal disorders of one sort or another. Too many of these victims of our "bigger is better" economic syndrome eventually developed serious intestinal trouble—chronic colitis, chronic constipation, rectal disorders and an endless assortment of digestive disorders that aggravated the lower belly. To relieve them, an endless assortment of pills and palliatives were popped into grim mouths during and after still grimmer meetings. Most of the "stomach settlers" did nothing but worsen their troubles by coating their bowels with chemical whitewash which sent them from extremes of diarrhea to constipation often by absorbing too much moisture. It never occurred to these pressured executives to give up the big lunches and the martinis and scotches that preceded them, or the drinks that unwound them at the end of the day, at quitting time and again before dinner. They took antacids, antihistamines and tranquilizers, all of which, when overused, contribute to various bowel disorders.

Instead of coping with the basic cause—the normal concerns of responsibility—by giving their gastrointestinal mechanism *less* to do, they gave their GI "machinery" more and more to do by loading up with too much food and drink, by taking antacids to put out the "burning sensation," by taking various kinds of tranquilizers and "calmer-downers" to cope with the hassle; and by eagerly running to the bar for that drink which, if the tranquilizers are still in their systems, can contribute directly to the coronary that probably will catch up with them in their prime years.

The title of this work, *Pre-Medicated Murder?*, is meant to imply that we help destroy our bodies by self-diagnosis and by treating ourselves with OTC remedies until, too late, we are driven to professional medical assistance.

This is seldom more true than in those cases where the gastrointestinal system is concerned. And still, reputable medical men agree that if we would employ a little common sense in our eating and working and recreational habits, the bulk of the problem never would trouble us—no pun intended!

Each specialist feels that his part of the human body is "a miraculous mechanism." And each is correct. The intricate design of the normal human body and the beautiful order of its operation is, indeed, a miracle; a miracle of evolution many believe—a mechanism perfectly adapted to its particular environment over hundreds of millions of years of "testing."

The basic thrust of the human mechanism is to "go right." A normally functioning body goes "wrong" when, through lack of understanding or carelessness, we abuse it. The great priority we give to commercial and career progress, and to the profit motive, has created a hostile environment for many of us. It is this constant push-pull battle of survival that upsets the normal functioning of much of our bodily mechanism—most especially the stomach and the bowels. (And that is not to ignore the most vital organ, the heart!)

How many times have you heard someone say, "I got so nervous I threw up?" Or, "Why is it I have to run to the 'can' before every big meeting?"

We knew a Broadway and film star who bemoaned the fact that "one minute before curtain time" she invariably had to "go."

Our "case of nerves" is not caused by our intestines and urinary mechanisms. It's the other way around. The "nervous trots" are an occupational ailment in most pressure professions. Anxiety or excitement, or both, transmit their disquieting messages through, among others, the complex vagi—the nerve network that controls the strength and frequency of the muscular contractions in the stomach and in our intestines; the organs that prepare the food and determine how efficiently it is digested; how quickly our stomaches empty; and how quickly, or slowly, the secondary digestive processes will take place in the 22 feet of our small intestines; and then how quickly, or slowly, the undigested or indigestible bulk, which is constantly having its fluids absorbed, moves on through the large intestine and into the "storage area" of our sigmoids; and finally down to the rectum and, hopefully, easily on out. (Like the foregoing sentence, a long, continuous process!)

No authority whose writings we've read, or to whom the authors have spoken personally, refuted the influence of emotion on this process. One doctor jokingly called it "the influence of mind over fecal matter."

The persuasiveness of this subliminal influence can be measured in dollars and cents. More than 750 proprietary preparations are sold over-the-counter to help move bowels. They offer us capsules, pills, fluids, solids to be chewed and solutions to be injected as enemas.

Each year we spend over $220 million on these preparations. And in most cases, they are dollars that could have been saved *if a little common sense knowledge had been gained and applied by the purchasers.* (We have purposely repeated that truth because it seems to escape so many of us!)

A simple explanation of the basic mechanism of the bowel may be helpful and reassuring.

There are four types of "movements" involving the stomach and intestines. They have two primary purposes: to churn or mix the contents of stomach and upper bowel and to propel the mixture along the 26 feet of the gastrointestinal tract where another system of impulses aids in ridding the body of the spent waste material.

Pendular movement is the motion of the longitudinal muscles in the intestine. The action of these long "up and down" muscles occurs at approximately 10 minute intervals. It is essentially a mixing movement.

Segmental movement involves contractions of the circular muscles and they occur at about the same intervals as pendular movement; they are also primarily mixing movements.

Peristaltic movement is a propelling motion. These movements travel along the intestinal tract toward the rectum. They seem to occur with varying frequencies, but physiologists feel that they happen "normally" at approximately one second apart. Their primary function is to move the contents through the small intestine. That process is said to take between 3½ to 4 hours in a normal gastrointestinal system.

Vermiform (worm-like) *movement* occurs chiefly in the large intestine, the colon, and is caused by the contraction of short segments of the colonic tissue. They are the sequential "bull dozer" movements in the colon, designed by nature to move larger masses of material which generally contain a significant amount of fluid.

By the time the contents of the bowel get to the transverse and descending colon and sigmoid or storage area just above the rectum, they are in a semisolid state in persons with normal bowel action.

At intervals of about six hours during the day, a very strong peristaltic action takes place that propels the contents along about one-third of the length of the colon. Apparently this activity is related to our eating habits. When we take on more food, the brain sends a signal to the gastrointestinal mechanism to "move out" the earlier intake. It is a case of "in one end and out the other," and the entire system is designed to function as a whole.

Actually, doctors say that the amount of fecal matter is what determines the frequency of a normal bowel movement. If we load our stomachs often we "get the urge." We humans modify that natural urge by various techniques of "toilet training" that are designed to accommodate our toilet habits to our life style.

Anyone who has been raised on a farm or ranch knows that when the animal population is fed, its members usually evacuate afterward. Their normal processes are not hampered by the need to catch the train or run to a meeting. They just *do what comes naturally,* as the song says. On ranches and farms, we very seldom find a constipated cow.

Ideally, nature would work the same way with us. But we don't let her. When we do not "answer nature's call" promptly, we frustrate the peristaltic process and the reflexes grow progressively weaker. If we persist in doing this, we get what some doctors call a "lazy bowel."

It is reassuring to know that chronic constipation is not generally due to organic malfunctions. Most often it is the result of ignoring nature's signals and then, later, attempting to "normalize" our bowels by the use of laxatives or inducing peristalsis, the more chronic becomes our problem because we are increasing our dependency upon outside remedies to do nature's work.

There is wide general misunderstanding of what consti-
tutes "normal" bowel movement patterns. Some people
have a normal evacuation pattern of twice a day; others,
once a day. Many perfectly normal persons move their bowels only three times a week. There are many documented
cases of persons who are quite normal and well who move
their bowels even less frequently. And in some, the pattern
may change from once a day to three or four times a week
with no vexatious consequences.

In his booklet, *You and Your Guts,* Dr. Clifford Hawkins,
a Fellow of the Royal College of Physicians in London, cites
medical claims that patients have gone up to eighty days
and longer while remaining "fit with good appetite and
plenty of energy."

One of the most prevalent old wives tales concerns the
"poisons" that allegedly are leached into our systems if we
do not open our bowels regularly each day.

"Sheer nonsense!" say physicians. There is no clinical evidence that anything happens to such people beyond a certain amount of discomfort which can be taken care of easily
and safely by a physician who will prescribe a mild laxative
or a carefully given enema.

Just as diahrrea may be caused by "undue pressure between the ears," as one physician put it, so can constipation
be caused by anxiety and change of routine. (More on this
in Chapter 7.)

It is not the purpose of this chapter to indict laxatives as
such, but merely to caution against abusing your gastrointestinal tract by overusing such preparations. Because a certain degree of self-medication is necessary, we are often
counselled by our physicians to take a mild laxative, if such-
and-such a conditon develops. Obviously, it must be a condition he does *not* regard as serious or dangerous.

Earlier we said that pharmaceutical houses have made the
task of buying a laxative easy by providing a choice of at least
750 different ones. But it does not follow that because the drug

store shelf is overcrowded with OTC laxatives one may close his eyes and pick a suitable remedy at random.

So-called OTC laxatives fall into several categories; and while any of them, used in moderation, may be acceptable for certain conditions in certain persons, all of them are far from safe for everybody.

Incidentally, the word "cathartic" generally means "purge" but common usage has tended to make the word a synomym for "laxative."

The ideal laxative, according to Dr. Roy C. Darlington, head of the Department of Pharmacy of Howard University, would be one that is nonirritating and nontoxic and acts only on the descending colon and the sigmoid colon. Moreover, it should produce one normally formed stool after which its effect would end.

So far as we could discover, no such specialized ideal laxative yet exists, although there are several that apparently limit their major activity to the colon. Among these would be stimulant anthraquinone preparations containing *cascara sagrada,* senna, rhubarb and aloe; *synthetic drugs* such as phenolphthalein, bisacodyl, danthron, oxyphenisatin acetate and oxyphenisatin; and among the *emollient fecal softeners,* mineral oils, poloxalkol and dioctyl sodium sulfosuccinate.

The *resinous laxatives* operate on both small and large intestine. Most common are agar, psyllium seeds (husks), sterculia (karaya gum), methylcullulose and sodium carboxymethylcellulose.

The foregoing bewildering array comprise the principal ingredients in most of the OTC laxatives sold under an equally bewildering array of trade names.

Since the Food and Drug Administration requires that all OTC drugs carry the list of ingredients on the label, it is possible to get a fair idea of what one is buying.

Your physician will know each of the ingredients and will know whether or not one or several of the various classes of laxatives are safe for your particular problem—if, indeed, he suggests an OTC remedy.

We would not presume, for this work, the function of a medical home advisory or even an encyclopedic collection of common OTC drugs. It is intended primarily as a "stitch in time" warning against the abuse of commonly used drugs that, for the most part, serve us well when used with discretion.

In the 100 preparations we checked in chain drugstores, the most widely used ingredient is phenolphthalein.

Questioning disclosed that this "workhorse" laxative ingredient, which is used alone and combined with other laxative agents, is a white crystaline substance that is a chemical compound of carbon, hydrogen and oxygen. It is soluble in alcohol; only slightly so in water.

In chemical laboratories, it is also a "workhorse" compound. When added to an alkali solution, the mixture turns red; when added to an acid solution, there is no color change. The color change not only happens in the chemist's flask, it also happens in one's intestine—if the feces are alkaline, as for instance, after the use of a soapy enema. If noted by the user, it may create some consternation!

Phenolphthalein can also be absorbed into the urinary system. If the urine happens to be alkaline also, and it often is, a person may find the fluid in the bladder is pink, and sometimes bright red. Unaware of the curious property, the user can get quite a shock. One physician reported a frantic patient who had run to the emergency ward of his local hospital swearing that he was bleeding internally. Actually, the phenomenon appears to be more spectacular than harmful, although it is possible that phenolphthalein may create allergies in some users.

A susceptible user may develop other side effects that are serious. A large dose or doses, taken regularly and frequently, have been known to cause severe diarrhea, skin eruptions and respiratory disorders. In extreme cases, cardiac distress and collapse have been reported.

Not so commonly used, but one whose action seems to resemble phenolphthalein, is oxyphenisatin acetate. It was found in several of the commonly used OTC laxatives.

Tests over a period of a year have shown that continued use of the drug may cause serious liver damage. This may be preceded by the symptoms of jaundice. One series of tests showed that continued overuse could duplicate the symptoms of hepatitis. The symptoms disappeared when the medicine was discontinued—and appeared again when the patient resumed using it.

The stimulant laxatives come mostly from natural sources. *Jalap* is extracted from a common Mexican flower that resembles the morning glory. It works on both the small and large intestine.

Cascara sagrada is derived from the bark of a tree native to many parts of the world, including the United States.

Senna belongs to the large and varied *Cassia* family which includes herbs, plants and trees. The sweet pulp of the cassia or senna pod has long been known as a purgative. Refined, it is a principal ingredient in a great number of proprietary laxatives.

Capsicum belongs to the nightshade family. It yields a strong stimulant that works on the entire gastrointestinal system. It is less used as a specific laxative than as a general "toner upper," but it is sometimes included with other natural laxatives.

Aloe also belongs to a large botanical family. The dried leaves and the juice extracted from the stems have long been used as a purgative. It is thought to be the "roughest" of the natural purgatives, and its ability to gripe the gut is second to none. And still it is found in several of the most popular "natural remedies," including one formulated especially for children. Most physicians urge that it be avoided.

The common saline laxatives have been listed earlier by their generic names. Few adults have not known the sudden and effective results achieved with *citrate of magnesia* (Milk of Magnesia)! These have been dependable purgatives. Most often they are "called for" (not prescribed) by doctors as part of the preliminary preparation for a gastrointestinal

X-ray examination. They are not deemed harmful with the exception of the sodium derivitives which can cause serious problems for a person with heart trouble.

Magnesium sulfate has been known to create problems for persons who have a depressed central nervous system, but the physicians interviewed were somewhat divided in their opinions as to the seriousness of such an effect.

Castor oil is considered one of the "natural laxatives," although the mere prospect of taking it has caused generations to do some unnatural things to avoid the experience. It works primarily on the small intestine, then hands its very positive results to the colon to dispose of. Its effect would seem to be the precise opposite of that of the "ideal" laxative mentioned earlier. Perhaps it is psychological; but to most people, it is the ultimate in distasteful remedies—even if it is labeled "tasteless."

Mineral oils are extremely common. Used by themselves or in combination with bulk forming substances, they are among the most frequently bought laxatives and "bowel conditioners."

For a long time, they were thought to be a benign blessing. But in recent years, research physicians have discovered that they inhibit the absorption of vitamins A and D. They also are said to have a deleterious effect on the absorption of calcium and phosphate, both critical "minerals" needed for a balanced physical machine.

Bulk-forming laxatives employ natural and semisynthetic substances that are generally cellulose derivitives. They form a soft mass or emollient jel in the intestine and ease the passage of the bowel contents by stimulating a natural reflex action that encourages peristalsis.

Except for the possibility that one may come to depend upon them unnecessarily and get the "bulk habit," they seem to have no bad effects. It is necessary, however, to increase one's fluid intake since they absorb fluid rapidly and could cause an impaction by "drying out" the intestinal contents. Used with plenty of water or fruit juices or other acceptable liquids, they work well and apparently do not interfere with the absorption of nutrients.

A final word about laxatives. There are some old remedies that still crop up in OTC laxatives. They are more apt to be found in small, out-of-the-way drug stores and general stores whose merchandise does not move rapidly.

They are highly irritating cathartics. As indicated, aloe is one. So is croton oil. Colocynth is another. Podophyllum qualifies in this category, and so does calomel, grandmother's old standby. Of these, calomel is deemed the most dangerous since its chemical name is *mercurous chloride*. If it remains in the bowel for an abnormally long time—a possibility if too small a dose is taken—it can have a very toxic effect. No physician interviewed would recommend calomel as a laxative. It has been replaced by far safer and more effective remedies.

And so, with no reluctance at all, we come to the end of our "incredible voyage" from the Adam's apple to the anus. It is only a 26-foot trip, but it is one that has created unbelievable human misery.

"Gut" is not a coarse word. It is a medically correct collective noun encompassing some of the most remarkable and durable machinery in the human body. If we give the gastrointestinal tract half a chance by not abusing it with too much food, too much drink (except water and acceptable substitutes) and too much of the 750 easily obtained, widely advertised OTC drugs, it will very likely see us through the four score and ten years classically allotted to us, plus a few more to boot.

7 Travelers' Diarrhea or "The Global Trots"

It might seem strange that such a subject would be included in a book titled *Pre-Medicated Murder?* In fact we had not planned such a chapter until Dr. Thaddeus Jones, our physician in Laguna Beach, began discussing the problems that can arise from self-medication and self-prescription in countries where many of the medicines ordinarily requiring a prescription in the United States may be bought over-the-counter.

Americans may have been superceded as "Champion Indefatigable World Travelers" by the newly affluent Japanese and West Germans. But millions of us still travel abroad each year. And we still suffer the same complaints and, too often, still bring the same diseases home with us because we do not listen to the common sense advice of our physicians, or because we listen to the ill-advised counsel of well-intentioned friends who pretend to have all the answers.

Far and away the most common ailment we are apt to contract abroad is known to physicians as "travelers diarrhea." It is seldom serious if the proper *simple* treatment is undertaken. And it is seldom contracted if a few simple precautions are heeded. Nearly every good travel agency and all overseas United States air carriers publish useful booklets and phamphlets that advise much the same precautions: Don't drink the tap water, drink bottled water or soft drinks. Don't chill them by dropping ice into them; the ice may be made of the tap water. Don't eat raw vegetables and fruits unless they are scrubbed and peeled. Don't overeat. Don't overdrink wines and other alcoholic beverages. Do rest before plunging into an itinerary (fat chance, if you're booked on the usual "breakneck" two week tour)!

All the foregoing is absolutely sound advice—which most of us do not follow to the letter. And then, when "Montezuma's Revenge" strikes in Mexico or the "Arabian Agonies" strike in the south of Spain and in North Africa and elsewhere around the Mediterranean, we smile as smugly as we can under the circumstances and reach for that little bottle of Entero-Vioform (an OTC in many countries) and begin popping pills, according to directions on the label, secure in the knowledge that it "always gets things under control."

Actually, it may. It has been used for years by travelers. Many physicians still recommend it. But a growing number of men, among them Dr. Thaddeus Jones who spends a great deal of time in Mexico and other foreign countries, now feel that *iodochlorhydroxyguin* (the generic name for Entero-Vioform) is probably more useful as a tongue-twister than as a "gut settler."

Recently the FDA came out with a recommendation that the remedy "not be given prophylactically" to travelers to protect them from diarrhea.

This warning was echoed in the *Physician's Bulletin* of the Orange County (California) Health Department, Volume 22, No. 7, March 27, 1972, by way of passing along a caution from the center for Disease Control in Atlanta, Georgia:

> Travelers' diarrhea occurs throughout the world, but it is most common where personal hygiene and sanitation are poor. The syndrome is characterized by diarrhea, often accompanied by vomiting, abdominal cramps, chills and low-grade fever. In most patients, the symptoms disappear in one to three days.
>
> The cause of travelers' diarrhea is uncertain. The disease is sometime attributed to unaccustomed or exotic foods and seasonings, but their involvement is doubtful. Specific microorganisms, i.e., *Shigella sp., Salmonella sp.* and *enteropathogenic Escherichia coli* are occasionally found in the stools of patients with travelers' diarrhea and recent studies suggest that toxin-producing and mucosal-penetrating strains of

E. *coli* may be the cause of this syndrome, but further study is necessary.

Iodochlorhydroxyguin (Entero-Vioform) has been used for many years to prevent travelers' diarrhea. Many tropical disease specialists believe that it is ineffective for this purpose. Recently, iodochlorhydroxyquin was implicated in Japan, Australia and Sweden as the cause of severe neurologic disease *subacute myloe-optic neuropathy,* a disease that erodes the sheath-like covering of the optic nerve. Therefore, until evidence is available to confirm or refute this association, physicians and travelers should be advised to refrain from prescribing or using iodochlorhy droxyquin (Entero-Vioform) to prevent travelers' diarrhea.

Travelers to areas where hygiene and sanitation are poor should be advised that the best way to prevent diarrhea is to eat only what can be peeled or has been cooked and to drink only boiled or bottled water, beverages that have been boiled, bottled carbonated soft drinks, bear and wine. Tap water used for tooth brushing and for ice in drinks can be a source of infection. However, tap water which is uncomfortably hot to the touch is usually safe. It may be used for oral hygiene and for drinking after cooling. If diarrhea does occur, it is usually short-lived; if it persists, a physician should be consulted.

Doctor Thaddeus Jones believes that fresh milk and cream may also be suspect in some foreign countries. In no case is it wise to buy food from street vendors. Cold meats (they may not have been refrigerated) can be dangerous and, we repeat because they are so tempting, those delicious appearing fresh salads. The vegetables, even if they have been washed thoroughly, quite probably were washed in city water—unless otherwise advertised.

Some of the newer hotels, particularly those operated by international chains, advertise their fresh fruits and vegetables as having been washed in "purified water." Personal experience in Mexico, Spain, Italy and the Caribbean, tends to bear out the reassurances. But in some parts of the world where vegetables are fertilized with "night soil" (human excrement), some very horrendous "bugs" can infiltrate the fibres and no amount of washing will get at them all.

Well-cooked meat is generally safe, even though it may have been plastered with flies hours earlier in the market. The same goes for well-cooked fresh fowl and fish.

However, there is a question as to how "fresh" an ocean fish is that has been trucked a hundred miles over the mountains to some interior city. Mobile refrigeration is not universally available in foreign countries. A fish that has begun to putrify on a truck cannot be "revived" simply by chilling it in the hotel or restaurant's refrigerator. But a clever chef can usually disguise putridity with a strong piquant sauce (*salsa picante*). After all, that is what the hot sauces and highly aromatic seasonings and spices were originally used for in the days before refrigeration. It is no coincidence that the "hottest" foods come from the hottest countries! "High" meat may not bother the natives; but unless one is used to it, it can make a traveler feel mighty "low"!

An important caution comes from Professor Howard C. Ansel, Head of the Department of Pharmacy at the University of Georgia. In a section on diarrhea remedies for the 1973 edition of *Handbook of Non-Prescription Drugs*, he wrote:

> It must be borne in mind that diarrhea is a symptom and that symptomatic relief must not be interpreted as a cure of the underlying cause. The judgment as to whether diarrhea is simple and uncomplicated and whether it should be treated symptomatically or with specific conjunctive therapy is that of the physician....

So what does one do medically to prevent travelers' diarrhea and other more serious infections?

Doctor Jones and a great many other physicians have come to have confidence in a preparation called *Lomotil* (Searle), the trade name for a compound called *diphenoxylate hydrochloride* plus *atropine sulfate*. It comes in both liquid and tablet form, the latter being preferred by travelers. It has a long "shelf life" in tablet form. That means that one may carry a supply almost indefinitely without risking a loss of effectiveness.

Although Dr. Jones will not claim that his personal use of Lomotil is infallible or for that matter even broadly effective, he and many of his patients, including the authors, take one tablet each day as a prophylactic. Neither the physician nor his author patients will testify to Lomotil's effectiveness as a prophylactic. But it does seem to work. However. it should be remembered that as frequent travelers who have learned "the hard way," we observe all those other "dos and don'ts" also.

It is possible to become accustomed to the food and drink of a foreign land if one spends sufficient time there. Then, upon returning home, a curious thing may happen—the person may get the "turistas" from eating and drinking his home town food and beverages!

Strangely enough, friends of ours from Mexico and Spain usually have a mild attack of travelers' diarrhea when they come to the United States. It varies from a very mild upset to a couple of miserable days before things sufficiently settle down in their gastrointestinal tracts.

If the diarrhea, nausea and fever persist for longer than three days, the traveler should immediately find a good doctor. That used to be difficult. In some areas of the world where tourists are now found in growing numbers, it still is. But generally speaking, an ailing person will find skilled medical help either in or associated with the best hotels. These establishments have a very important public relations stake in seeing that their guests are well taken care of in case of an emergency. If one should require hospitalization, there are usually several to choose from in the large population centers. Most Latin-American and European countries are equipped with the latest developments and with personnel trained in their use.

Should the hotel not be able to locate a dependable physician, it is possible to join a service called *Intermedic*. When one joins, a directory is provided giving the names and addresses of associated English-speaking physicians in nearly every important city in the world. These men are properly qualified by the Intermedic examiners. By calling the Intermedic office in the large cities of the United States, one may get current enrollment and other charges (prices are quoted in U.S. dollars). Or one may write to Intermedic, Inc., 777 Third Avenue, New York, N.Y. 10017. The organization's roster of officers and medical board reads like a "Who's Who" in American medicine.

We asked Dr. Thaddeus Jones about some of the other commonly used remedies for the effects of travelers' diarrhea. "Kaopectate works. But it is not a preventive medicine. It acts like a blotter," he explained. "It soaks up the excess fluid associated with diarrhea."

We asked about kaolin preparations containing paregoric (tincture of opium).

It can be effective in reducing discomfort (and) cramps but again, it is not a preventive. An older physician friend of mine who regularly went on fishing trips to Mexico used to dose himself with ten drops of paregoric once a day. He swore it helped him avoid trouble. I suspect though that what it did was calm him down a bit. Just the excitement (and) the anticipation of a good trip can be enough to upset the gastrointestinal tract. I think today we probably have better preparations to take care of that contingency. But paregoric is a reliable and useful medication.

Doctor Jones reminded us that since it contains opium, it must be obtained on a special triplicate prescription which places a strict limit on refills. In several foreign countries, however, we were able to buy paregoric as an over-the-counter drug.

Without becoming a "crock" about it, there are some things that a person can do to ensure a safe and happy trip from a health point of view.

A practical first aid kit containing a soluble aspirin; a mild nasal spray (important for air travelers); some adhesive bandages for minor cuts and scratches; a mild antacid preparation, preferably a tablet; and of course, Lomotil or some other preparation that your personal physician has found helpful. But remember, these do not cure. They merely supply relief and comfort while the "bug" runs its course.

We say "bug" but many doctors, including Dr. Jones, feel that travelers' diarrhea may also involve a viral infection. That would explain why none of the antibiotics seem to help. As we have seen before, the viruses that cause a wide range of illnesses and diseases are not affected by the so-called "miracle drugs."

Depending upon your destination, there are certain other mandatory and optional precautions that should be taken.

One's small pox vaccination should be checked to make certain it is still effective. If one is needed, three weeks should be allowed for it to "take" and calm down. If one is getting a repeat or a booster, only ten days would be required to make certain it is effective.

The vaccinations required vary from country to country. The Department of Health, Education and Welfare publishes annually, a booklet updating these requirements. It is known as *Public Health Service Publication No. 384,* U.S. Department of Health, Education and Welfare, Public Health Service. It may be obtained by writing to Superintendent of Documents, U.S. Government Printing Office, Washington, D.C. 20402. In the past, the price has been $.40. Chances are your personal physician will have one available or have access to one. Since a wise traveler will have a good checkup before leaving, all this information can be obtained during the office visit. If you are going to take an extensive trip, a freighter trip for instance, during which many ports in many countries will be visited, your physician may recommend vaccinations or medication for a wide range of possible infections and diseases, including cholera, typhoid, yellow fever, hepatitis and measles. For *any* trip, he may recommend polio and tetanus immunization.

In short, what you will need depends upon where you are going. If you think there is a possibility that you'll depart from your original itinerary and get off the beaten track, try to prepare for that too. "Off the beaten track" is where one is most likely to need help and is least likely to get it! So, if you go, "Vaya con Dios" and a lot of good common-sense medical advice. If you do, your most precious slides will be the ones you took with your camera, not the ones the laboratory technician put under the microscope to find out what you caught!

Doctor David R. Nalin, a Johns Hopkins University researcher and Dr. Stephen Richardson, a microbiologist with Bowman-Gray Medical College in Winston-Salem, North Carolina, believe they are on the track of a vaccine that will knock out travelers' diarrhea.

A news story carried in the Los Angeles *Times*, Sunday, April 8, 1973, indicated that a new anticholera serum also seems to be effective against *E. coli toxin*, one of the prime suspects. If true, the researchers feel it may also prevent *E. coli* diarrhea. However, like so many promising new medical discoveries, it is not available yet. Neither is it likely to be soon.

8 Mouthwash or Hogwash?

In 1972, Americans spent $240,580,000 on various proprietary "mouth washes."* That is just short of a *quarter of a billion* hard-earned dollars spent for preparations that are acknowledged as useful in maintaining the general tone of healthy oral cavities but are universally thought to be of little or no value if they are used for the prevention and cure of the "sore throat" associated with the common cold.

In Chapter 5, we saw that none of the topical remedies available, either over-the-counter or by prescription, are specific preventives or cures for *viral-initiated* infections anywhere in the respiratory system.

Preparations containing proved germicidal agents in varying strengths are useful in the general oral "house-cleaning" process. Depending upon how they are applied—gargled, douched or sprayed—they kill varying numbers and varieties of germs, most of which are normally present in the mouth and throat.

In a matter of minutes after we are born, indeed, seconds after the first protesting squawk following that first spank on the bottom, we begin offering shelter to some of the germs that will take up residence in our mucous membranes and reside there until life ends, and then some!

They have familiar and often fearsome names: *streptococcus, pneumococcus, staphylococcus, lactobacillus* are among the most common. They live and multiply by the millions in the folds and crevices of the mucous membrane

*Drug Topics, September 25, 1972.

and they congregate on the smooth, relatively easy-to-get-at surfaces too.

Effective germicidal agents—the phenol compounds, the two basic types of alcohol, some iodine compounds and hydrogen peroxide solutions—can reduce the germ population superficially. But as we have seen, they are useless against infections caused by the viruses that also normally inhabit our oral cavities.

Our natural defense mechanisms usually keep these "bug" populations living in a state of static balance with each other and with our entire system. Not all germs have the same life span. Some are hatched and live for only a few hours before our natural defenses, or other bacteria, kill them. Others live for several days, for a week or a month, and some authorities say, still others appear to live with us for all of our days.

Dangerous "outside and indigenous invaders" can get a foothold and a war can start if something happens to disrupt the delicate "balance of power." We say that we are subject to infection when our "resistance is lowered." That can mean many specific things in many parts of the body and there can be many causes—improper diet, not enough rest and improper medication.

In the oral cavities, these "spelunking" viruses and bacteria can burrow deep into the crevices that are present throughout the entire respiratory system. There, safe from the superficial topical attacks of germicidal agents in commercial gargles and mouthwashes, they can "dig in and establish a beach head" from which they can invade the entire system.

Some of the viruses seem to enter the blood stream and go exploring until they find a weakened area. It might be an injured area or one in which we, having diagnosed our own "sore throat" as of no consequence, proceed to upset the balance of power by killing some of the friendly bugs that are a part of our physiological defense mechanism.

Recently a considerable segment of the medical profession has made a complete reverse on the matter of taking out tonsils and adenoids as a "routine procedure."

There is persuasive evidence that nature designed our spongy, limphoid tissues—the palatine and the pharyngeal tonsils (adenoids)—as catch-alls for potentially harmful bacteria. It is thought by many doctors that so-called "tonsilitis," unless it becomes chronic, is simply nature's way of warning us that we've been invaded. If the battle is contained and won in the tonsils and adenoids, there is less likelihood that the infection will spread to other parts of the respiratory tract; so the theory goes. This point of view is neither new nor unanimous. When tonsilectomies were first undertaken back in the late nineteenth century, most of the "old family doctors" were outraged at what they called "this mutilation of the voice box"! They were convinced that everything, including the veriform appendix, was "put into us by God for a good and sufficient reason and ought not to be 'butchered out' like the testes of shoats."

There was a great deal of controversy, even over an inflamed appendix. When an appendix burst and peritonitis set in, the mortality rate was high, even after the advent of antisepsis and drainage techniques pioneered by the English surgeon, Joseph Lister (1827-1912), and the use of more sophisticated compounds of chloroform first used as an anesthetic by Sir James Simpson in 1848.

Pursuing the logic that if a life could be saved by cutting out an inflamed appendix then, in the case of an acutely inflamed tonsil or adenoid, the same happy result might be achieved, early surgeons lost many patients. It was not until very late in the nineteenth century that it was generally understood that tonsilectomies were best undertaken during quiescent periods when no inflamation was present. And now it would appear that the "circle will come full" and the old philosophy will gain many new adherents.

All of this is related, indirectly, to our proclivity for self-diagnosis and medication. It has never been a wise thing to do when carried to extremes. Alexander Pope said "a little learning is a dangerous thing," and Thomas Huxley asked, much later, if there is any man who possesses so much knowledge that he is "out of danger."

Most physicians will confess that so far as the medical profession is concerned, there is no man who knows so much that he is beyond the danger of making an imperfect diagnostic judgment. If that is not contested in the profession, certainly it should not be contested by the laity. And still every day scores of patients finally are driven to see physicians because the "sore throat" they thought could be handled casually with OTC remedies does not respond.

One hardly needs to be reminded of the high incidence of venereal disease in these sexually permissive times. Syphilis, once an endemic disease, is now epidemic in many areas. The particular tragedy is that it is striking young people who feel that since our new morality seems to condone if not approve indescriminate love-making, they are somehow immune. "If it isn't evil, you won't catch anything," said a sixteen-year-old girl in a Southern California free clinic. A carrier, she was suspected of having infected at least a dozen young men.

It was a sore throat that brought her to the attention of the young physicians who volunteer a certain number of hours each week treating the indigent "street people." A young man came in with a persistent "canker sore" on his tongue. One look and the physician identified it as a chancre, a primary lesion. Under questioning, the lad identified the girl who was asked to come in. Two other young male companions had developed "sore throats" that were caused by chancres around the tonsil sites. The girl herself was developing a lesion at the corner of her mouth. All had been treating themselves with "mouthwashes" and "gargles." One of the young men had been taking a strong infusion of ginseng tea for his sore throat because "the lady in the health food store told me that it would build up my sex drive by building up my system and if my system was strong the sore throats would go away."

In time, the infection was arrested in these young people by intensive courses of "miracle drugs" administered by the physicians. They also administered some "sound advice" and an elementary lesson in prophylaxis.

Oral lesions are often a sign of leukemia in its early stages. Pernicious anemia may often manifest itself by oral lesions also. That sore throat may be a strep infection. If not properly treated, the infection can cause rheumatic fever and nephritis—a dangerous kidney disorder.

Mononucleosis, at its onset, is often mistaken for a common sore throat. One hardly needs to elaborate on the folly of attempting to determine the subtle differences in these similar symptoms without a great deal of specialized knowledge and the benefits of modern lab technology.

Doctors pride themselves on practicing "good medicine." That means they try to employ conservative, logical medical practices. Most doctors will confess that a lot of the work they do entails treating symptoms. But the point is this—they are trained to recognize those symptoms and to differentiate between those with only subtle differences, so subtle that the average person could never in a thousand years tell the dangerous difference between a staph infection in the throat and a syphilitic lesion or chancre in the area where a tonsil once was.

On a less serious level, it is possible that the protracted use of broad-spectrum antibiotics given to "shotgun" an infection the doctor is not absolutely certain of, or given to get at a multiple bacterial infection, may cause an allergic reaction that can be confused with a sore throat.

Usually the effect will disappear with a change or withdrawal of the medication. But again, one of the most commonly shared medicines are the antibiotics. Hardly a person who has bought the miracle drugs on prescription can resist "recommending" this one or that to a friend who is apparently suffering from the same ailment. And too often the well-intentioned samaritan will just happen to have a few capsules left in the refrigerator or in the medicine cabinet. If hell is paved with good intentions, then for sure a great many hospital rooms are peopled by patients who borrowed medication from a friend. "Harp on that theme!" said Dr. Murray Hoffstein of New York's Mt. Sinai Hospital. "It is a common and very harmful practice."

To sum up: many of the commercial gargles and mouthwashes can be useful in maintaining good oral hygiene. But it can be very dangerous to diagnose your own throat ailment as just a "common sore throat" and attempt to treat the symptoms yourself with these OTC preparations.

Many dangerous, *potentially fatal diseases,* in their early stages, masquerade as one of the symptoms of a "common cold." It is worth remembering that the National Academy of Sciences, National Research Council is recorded as saying, "There is no convincing evidence that any medicated mouthwash, used as a part of a daily hygiene regimen, has therapeutic advantage over a physiologic saline solution or even water."

So, it must be apparent that the possibilities for misjudging symptoms by self-diagnosis are legion and such a mistake may lead to serious and perhaps even fatal illnesses.

In tests it has been shown that alcohol is one of the most efficent germicidal agents. There are many types of alcohol, the most common being ethyl. In vitro (test tube) experiments have shown that ethyl alcohol is probably the most efficient germ killer. But not in the concentrations found in most OTC gargles and mouthwashes.

A series of tests run by scientists of the Food and Drug Administration show that a 70 percent concentration of ethyl alcohol is the most effective in killing certain common germs found in the oral cavity. But even a powerful 100 proof alcoholic drink has only 50 percent alcohol. The 70 to 90 percent concentrations of alcohol took as long as one minute to kill certain dangerous throat lodged bacteria. Even if most of us gargled or sprayed our throats for as long as that, there seems little chance that the fairly low (0.5 to 25 percent) concentrations of alcohol in some popular mouthwashes would do much good in the case of a serious condition.

None of the physicians interviewed would state categorically that the popular OTC products available in most drug stores and supermarkets would do more than assist in the basic oral hygiene every person should undertake each morning and evening to stop the growth of bacteria in the decaying food particles inevitably left behind after the usual "lick and a promise" brushing.

The FDA is presently undertaking an in-depth reevaluation of the principal proprietary medicines. They are breaking them down into twenty-five main categories. Each of these separate divisions will be thoroughly evaluated and decisions will be made as to the validity of claims on their labels and the accuracy of the ingredient listings.

There is a strong feeling in the FDA that many of the claims and ingredient lists may be misleading to the average customer, if indeed, the person takes the trouble to read them. We are so motivated by advertising to ask for or reach for a popular brand name that we think the name is enough. We can trust the manufacturer; his word is gospel. As the song from *Porgy and Bess* reminds us, "It ain't necessarily so...."

In the sixteenth century, a German botanist named Euricius Cordus wrote a warning in his book on contemporary drugs: "Through sheer ignorance a considerable portion of the jars and drawers and packets in the drug shops are falsely labeled."

In this respect, the Food and Drug Administration suspects that we have not progressed very far in four hundred years!

9 The Whole Tooth (and Nothing but the Truth)

In *Much Ado About Nothing,* Shakespeare wrote, "there was never yet a philosopher that could endure the toothache patiently."

As with much of the Bard of Avon's fundamental observations, most of us are not disposed to argument. And the memory of the toothache will certainly throb through literature and folklore for as long as man recalls the deepest of his miseries.

To a student of *minutiae personae,* the real miracle of the Declaration of Independence and the Constitution of the United States of America is not that it was written by such young men, but that it was written by men of any age who appeared to suffer chronically from toothache! And what about the Revolution and Yorktown, and Cornwallis and General George Washington on his white charger—with his "painless steel" false teeth? Undoubtedly Cornwallis had poor teeth (the English and their mutton, you know). Could it be possible then that our independence from their George III's British Empire was really won because our George W. had the foresight to rid himself of his malefic molars and the distraction they created?

Between the time young Todd Lincoln might have barged into the Oval Room to holler, "Look Pop, only one tooth!" and those commercials where contemporary professional nippers burst into board meetings shouting, "Look Dad, only one *cavity!*" lies a lot of lore, a lot of research, but strangely enough, few answers to the fundamental question, "How

are we going to get people turned on to proper dental hy
giene early enough to preserve the teeth they have
inherited?"

Those "supper-time" commercials showing happy dent
ure wearers munching corn-on-the-cob, candy apples, blue-
berry muffins and cherry tarts—foods guaranteed to either
tilt or tint most false teeth—are aimed at some 23 million
Americans who either inherited hopelessly poor teeth and
lost them or who did not take the few minutes of daily
hygienic time that could have saved their teeth for some
time at least.

The figure represents 10 percent of our population as of
the 1970 census. It also represents "economic teeth" when
one considers that the manufacturers of products for the
cleaning and maintenance of dentures are something on the
order of a $220 million dollar market.

Dental problems in early years parlay into big earnings
for dentists and drug companies as the years wear on. Cavities are said to cause most of our problems prior to age
forty. But after forty, periodontal troubles—pyorrhea, trench
mouth, gingivitis and a brace of other stubborn troubles—
account for fifteen to twenty times more expense and agony
than simple decay caused by dental caries. Most family
dentists, pedodontists, orthodontists and endodontists agree
that it is possible to dramatically reduce these serious
dental troubles—some of which lead to extended bone surgery—by doing something as simple as brushing your teeth
at night with a warm solution of common table salt and a
pinch of soda, a precaution that many an old pioneer grandmother urged to avoid the agony of an aseptic extraction by
the town barber.

It is a safe assumption also that those pioneer grand-
fathers, having survived the extraction, thought that a "little
more whiskey" disinfected the raw socket. As a matter of
fact, from long remembered personal childhood observation, we also thought that to be true. Superficially, at least,
the topical application of 100 proof psychoactive "white
lightening" was every bit as efficient (or inefficient) as any

of the fanciest mouthwashes and oral antiseptics on the market today—and some cheaper too!

The injunction, "Brush your teeth three times a day and see your dentist twice a year," has been modified somewhat. Now many dentists feel that while children cannot take too many precautions to ensure a good dental "start," adults really need to do a *thorough* cleaning job only once a day, preferably before going to bed.*

For a decade or more, we've heard the pros and cons of the fluoride story. What seems to be emerging is very interesting. There is little doubt that fluoridization of the city water has actually resulted in a great improvement in the dental health of children.

In the 2,836 communities that add one part per million of fluoride to their drinking water, there is an *incontestable decrease* in the incidence of dental caries among children.

Evidence notwithstanding, a number of alarmed ultra-conservative parents (and a lot of childless taker-uppers-of-causes) have raised not-so-merry hell at city hall when the plan has been proposed. Often they've been successful. But despite their sincere concerns, the scientific evidence is preponderantly in favor of fluoridization.

Chicago was the first major U.S. city to legalize fluoridization. Surveys indicate a 50 percent *decrease* in tooth decay among the city's school children. This translates into an annual savings to parents of some $20 million annually in dental bills,** to say nothing of the avoidance of human misery.

Doctor W. E. Schiefer of San Diego, President of the California Dental Association, found the same result in West Coast cities with fluoridated water supplies. Speaking to the Orange County Dental Society in September 1973, he revealed that one of the largest insurance companies selling prepaid dental insurance is now offering a 50 percent reduc-

---

*For this many dentists now recommend a *soft*, nylon bristled brush whose tips have been rounded so as not to damage or traumatize the sensitive gum tissue along the tooth margins.

**The authors have first-hand evidence of this benefit in their Chicago-reared and educated daughter and her contemporaries!

tion in premiums if the children who are insured have lived in fluoridated communities for three years or more.

Direct applications of fluoride solutions to the teeth of children in communities where fluoridization is not permitted—or has not yet been considered—is helpful. But there is a little disagreement that the best way is to let the *one-part-in-a-million* make its way through the interior structure of the growing tooth, thus immunizing it against dental decay "from the inside out" so to speak.

The effectiveness picture for adults' teeth is less clear; however, there is strong evidence that it does help to maintain strong bones.

While there is some *evidence* that the direct application of fluoride solutions is occasionally helpful in patients still under thirty, most dentists tend to minimize its effectiveness.

At this point, the adult must rely on another procedure. Primarily, it will consist of careful dental hygiene: regular brushing and flossing; rinsing with a gentle salt solution, or with a mouthwash if one prefers; and if possible, using one of the water jet devices to dislodge food particles from between the teeth and under the margins of the gums.

There is a growing feeling that the old up-and-down brushing technique that we've been enjoined to use for years is not the best way to go about it. Also, many dentists now feel that the electric toothbrush is superior to the hand driven models because it manages a thousand strokes or more a minute to the 180 or so that most vigorous brushers manage, usually with some damage to their gums if they use a hard split-bristled brush. The latest thinking now calls for a soft brush and a new approach to the brushing motion, with or without the electric aid.

The brush should be placed against the teeth at a 45-degree angle with the bristles pressed against the margins of the gums. Then, instead of the vigorous up-and-down driving and scrubbing, the brush should be oscillated in a subtly circular motion to make certain that the bristles "scoop" gently at the edges of the gum line where plaque forms and that they penetrate between the teeth.

A dentifrice should be used. But which one? Apparently there are a number of them on the market designed for special purposes. Some are for general cleaning and polishing. Some are for tender or sensitive teeth and gums and others are primarily brighteners that usually contain a high percentage of some abrasive ingredient. Many dentists regard these with reservations. "Your teeth can't be made any whiter than nature made them," said Dr. M. Joe Brockman who, in addition to a large general practice, is a member of the teaching staff at the University of Southern California School of Dentistry in Los Angeles. "There is a real chance of eroding the enamel if they are used to extremes," he added.

The problem is not so much of "brightness" as of cleanliness. Doctor Brockman believes the newest soft brush technique described in the foregoing is not doing as well as most dentists anticipated.

> It isn't that the brushing technique is wrong or that the accepted brands of toothpaste are not effective. There is much evidence that they are. The real trouble is the problem we dentists have in motivating our patients. It is very difficult to get them to take the time and effort needed to properly clean their teeth. Even when we tell adults that one good cleaning just before bedtime will help greatly, they seem reluctant to take even that small precaution. There is just so much a dentist can do in that direction. It is a problem of on-going education. We do not stop trying.

What Dr. Brockman is saying, inferentially, is that human nature hasn't changed; we insist on believing that "dental disaster" will happen to the *other* person. We will train our children to brush and rinse, but we "busy" adults seem to be waiting for some sort of an "instant" remedy that will allow us to swish a little fluid through our teeth, expel it and smile at that medicine cabinet mirror to admire our "rinso white," "squeaky clean" teeth; and all done in fifteen seconds or less! "No way," say the dentists. There is a possibility that some day we may be able to ward off dental caries with a vaccine much as we guard against smallpox, polio and other epidemic diseases. But don't wait. While early experiments are "promising," they are not yet at the hopeful stage.

A number of culprits lie in wait to attack our teeth. Those bits of food that lodge between the teeth and just under the margins of the gums. The sugars that we Americans ingest in such huge quantities, which may also contribute to illnesses far more serious than tooth decay. And, most important of all, a gluey, gooey, invisible substance called "dental plaque" that provides a veritable condominium for bacteria that interact to ferment the sugars and change them to acids that "etch" the enamel and open the way for the decay process.

There is no way that one can keep plaque off teeth, even for a short period of time. Clean it off and it will start to form again in minutes. Our saliva helps by depositing the new batch in a microscopic layer at the base of our teeth along the gum line. Once the plaque starts, the foundation is laid for a new colony of "bugs" who will happily feed on residual sugars in the mouth, spew out their acid, die and turn into flinty bits of a substance called "tartar." With dental plaque, eternal vigilance is the price of freedom from dental decay. Dental plaque is the foundation upon which the tartar builds. It is the primary culprit, the hardest to detect and the one that needs the most persistent pursuit.

Since dental plaque is so hard to see, a dye product has been developed that stains the plaque a bright pink. It is harmless and when it has been brushed away, the plaque is gone too. But only for the time being.

The "dye marker" pills intrigue children. They take them, watch the little patches of plaque turn red, then go after them with vigor until they disappear. It is a big help, a fine motivator. But if these youngsters are using fluorides in one form or another—in their drinking water, applied topically to the teeth by their dentists or through the use of one of the ADA approved dentifrices containing caries inhibitors—the most important part of their protection is already under way.

It is really the adults who need to use the "little pink pills" to stain the plaque since, as we have seen, it is universally believed in the dental profession, *and it has not yet been disproved,* that fluorides do little or no good in preventing dental decay in grownups. In short, there is no substitute for a good cleaning.

The alternative is a lot of expensive dentistry with a good likelihood that sooner or later we'll join that 10 percent or more who will end up wearing dentures. To paraphrase the late Dorothy Parker, "Folks who wear dentures have darned bad adventures."

Those little rubber tips on some toothbrushes, or smooth, round toothpicks, plastic massage gadgets, balsa wood "matches" and a number of other especially designed little "picking" devices can be helpful in combating decay and forestalling the periodontal diseases that often result. Anything that tends to clean the inner tooth surfaces and the gum margins gently, without traumatizing (shocking) them is helpful. But the first line of defense is to get after that placque.

Because we are assailed on all sides by the superiority claims of various dentifrices, there is a natural skepticism in most of us—thanks to advertising.

Recently, however, several popular toothpastes have been able to substantiate their claims that their "special ingredients" are effective in combating tooth decay. Their independently undertaken tests were examined by the American Dental Association's Council on Dental Therapeutics, were found to be "acceptable" and were listed in *Accepted Dental Therapeutics* and given the right to display the official seal.

Crest containing stannous fluoride and Colgate with MFP (sodium monofluorophosphate) were judged "effective decay-preventive dentifrices." Preliminary tests on Gleem II containing fluoride indicate a similar advantage for that product. So it seems that in some cases we need not be skeptical of those handsome young TV "scientists in their white coats earnestly flashing their bound reports. Apparently they have something there—for the kiddies, at least.

Dental opinion is divided about the advisability of using such decay preventives in combination with a water fluoridization program. In the main, the dentists interviewed took the position that "it probably doesn't hurt." They were more conservative about combining the topical office application of fluorides with the day-to-day drinking water program. Most of them said it seemed unnecessary to risk the chance of toxicity by doing both.

Diet is a major factor in dental health. Many dentists, including Dr. Brockman, feel that most adults today are getting too much phosphorous and not enough calcium in their diets. There is some divergence of opinion about the ratio of calcium to phosphorous. The concensus seems to be about five parts of calcium to one of phosphorous. Some said six to one.

Milk and milk products are still a primary source of calcium for those who have "no trouble" with milk. For those who do, doctor will often prescribe calcium tablets in carefully regulated dosages. Self-prescription of calcium via drug or health food OTC products can be very hazardous, especially in the presence of joint diseases. If one suspects a calcium deficiency, the safest thing is to ask a medical doctor or dentist who will recommend tests to make certain.

It is not the purpose of this book to find some "deadly danger" in every chapter. And still, in dealing with the human body, even in dentistry, it is not safe to assume that work on one's teeth is an "isolated project" with little or no relation to the rest of the body.

While it is true that for most of us, the routine dental work holds little or no danger of anything more serious than physical and financial discomfort, there are some patients who can actually be risking their lives when they go to their dentists for extensive work.

A person who has had *rheumatic heart disease* and goes to the dentist and does not inform him, either personally or through the questionnaire that should be filled out by every new patient, is taking a grave risk.

Most U.S. dentists demand such a questionnaire. But what if the patient—especially an older patient—simply "forgets" to put down that ailment of years ago? Very simply, such a patient is in great danger of developing a disease called *subacute bacterial endocarditis*.

At New York's Mt. Sinai Hospital, Dr. Murray Hoffstein said,

> The manipulation of a tooth can develop into a serious disease.
> For instance maloclusion could impinge on carious teeth and a
> subacute bacterial endocarditis may result. It is extremely dan-
> gerous. It has a grave prognosis and can result in death in a
> short period of time. A dentist who is aware of the previous
> condition will always insure his patient's recovery with prophy-
> lactic antibiotic therapy.

It is worth repeating that most modern dentists demand a
properly filled out questionnaire revealing the patient's past
illnesses. Also, if they are not entirely satisfied with the
writing after "sizing up" the new patient, they may resort to
additional verbal questioning.

But what about the patient who has had some emergency
work done overseas while on a holiday tour and develops
the disease on the way home? Such a patient, the emergency
doctors observe, are "in need of all our skills and all of their
family's prayers!"

The dental health outlook a generation hence is hopeful
indeed. It would be phenomenally bright if preventive dentistry were universally practiced in our schools—the regular
ingestion of carefully fluoridated drinking water, or regular
topical treatment with fluoride preparations by visiting
dentists and the cultivation of regular and effective dental
prophylactic habits.

That is asking a lot of our coke-guzzling, candy-munching
youngsters. It is even asking a lot, apparently, of our local
and regional PTA groups and politicians who too often mistrust the scientific evidence that fluoridation helps and re-
fuse to initiate school-wide dental health programs. Adults
and parents don't hesitate ten seconds to take advantage of
preventive procedures if a polio or typhoid or measles epidemic threatens. But tooth decay has been "epidemic" for
generations and remains so in many areas, through the prejudice, timidity and (perhaps, or) disinterest of adults who
could demand action and get it, at all levels.

Many dentists, Dr. Brockman among them, admit that the biggest criticism of their profession stems from the fact that it was slow to initiate research on prevention. "But we are hard at it now," he said, "and the ideal our profession is aiming for is perfect prophylaxis. In USC alone, there are a dozen programs underway, heading toward that goal."

The authors know from inquiry that many such programs are in full swing in dental schools here, in Canada and in England. One of these days, hopefully before Junior is a parent telling his own offspring that he wished he'd listened to his parents, the perfect dental prophylaxis regimen will be established. Nobody believes it will come soon.

Meantime, too many of today's children will grow up missing or abusing the advantages we presently can enjoy and will have misadventures with their dentures.

One of the simplest and most common "good tooth insurance" practices can be undertaken when children are losing their "baby teeth." For centuries it has been Daddy's prerogative to tie the string to the tooth, make all sorts of diversionary noises and yank the loose member out. Except for a little mild outrage that it didn't really hurt after all, there was little danger in the process, and some reward if the tooth was put under the pillow. The trouble is, the process stops with this home extraction—and it should not.

Underneath some of those first teeth are the permanent teeth that, hopefully, will see us through the years of our lives. Under ideal circumstances, they will come in at the proper time and in the proper places. But often they do not. Inherited facial structure may be an influence. Eating habits may modify the natural course of growth. So this is the time to seek the counsel of the pedodontist, the specialist in childhood tooth problems, who can do some very simple things to ensure the appearance of straight, strong, properly spaced permanent teeth.

One of the simplest of these procedures is to fit the child with spacers that will ensure room for the new tooth in the young jaw. There are few more satisfying experiences than to watch the results of modern preventive dentistry on one's own child. No dollars ever spent on prevention will bear more satisfactory or long term dividends.

The alternatives, while effective, are certainly not pleasant.

Every once in a while some popular family magazine will run an article on progress in tooth replacement. Generally they are surveying the research being done into the possibility of implanting an artificial tooth (or teeth) into the jawbone in such a way that they will become an integral part of the anatomy, much as the original tooth was.

So far, little of the experimental work seems to be truly promising. Recently a substance called *vitreous carbon* appeared. It seems to offer some encouragement. Experiments on patients have not run long enough to be definitive. So far, the implant procedure is only 50 percent effective, on a short term basis. Dentists say that they will not begin to consider the implant technique "practical" until better than 80 percent of the applications are successful, and over a much longer time span.

The problem is to make the artificial tooth "take hold" in the jawbone. From that central problem others proliferate. To do that the tooth must be anchored. It is not practical to attempt that mechanically since the jawbone is porous and screws and clamps can't be secured firmly. The motion may cause irritation, infection and rejection.

One alternative would be the development of a cement-like substance that would "stick" to both the vitreous carbon tooth and the living jawbone without becoming toxic to the latter.

By nature, researchers, are both persistent and optimistic. The chances are that they'll put together the effective combination before universal preventive dental hygiene becomes a fact and the need for artificial teeth mercifully has been eradicated by the benevolent science of medicine and dentistry.

In the meantime, when one surveys the products and procedures presently available to help us "hold the health line," it seems foolish to do less than investigate the possibilities with an open mind. Medical and pharmaceutical research is not perfect; but in the main it is dedicated and entirely responsible. From these efforts have come boons that have increased man's lifespan by 30 percent in little more than a century. It seems foolish to wait for the miracle cure. The "bugs" that erode our teeth are not waiting. In the meantime, there is much we can do to slow down their evil work while, at the same time, ensuring ourselves and our children of many more trouble-free hours of daily life. A researcher may wish that it would all happen faster. But one cannot help but be grateful to those dedicated men and women—medical doctor, dentists, biologists and chemists—whose lives are in direct contradiction to the generally unjust charge that they pursue their careers to "get rich" when, in fact, they are pursuing their research to enrichen us. If they were disposed to waste their time with an "eye for an eye, tooth for a tooth" philosophy, they might, with much justice, charge most of us with being stupid or at the very least, short-sighted, for not practicing the preventive procedures they have already tested and proved.

10 Antacids and the "Gas House Gang"

He was a good friend of ours, a happy go-lucky, talented man with a wonderful career and a family who returned his love. He smoked a little, drank almost not at all (a ceremonial cup on birthdays and anniversaries) and ate moderately. For years he had been troubled from time to time by "a touch of gastritis"; a little burning here," he would say, pointing to his mid-chest. Then he would take one of his favorite "alkalizers" or "bromide" settlers, feel better and go on his useful, merry way.

We found him unconscious one day, in his own garden. He lived for a week in intensive cardiac care. The family agreed to an autopsy "for what good it may do others."

The autopsy showed two things: our friend had been suffering from *angina pectoris,* apparently for some time, and the medication he had been taking for his "touch of gastritis" had either caused or had aggravated a serious peptic ulcer.

Later, the pathologist said the lining of our friend's stomach was literally "riddled" with small perforations apparently caused by undissolved particles of potassium bromide. "Even without the cardiac condition, this was a very sick man," he commented.

How could a mild heart condition of several years standing be confused with hyperacidity? Quite simply, say physicians. There are a number of serious diseases whose early symptoms may actually mimic the pain usually associated with the discomfort we commonly call "gastritis." They are difficult to pin down.

To the layman, gastritis is a sort of catch-all term that is not medically accurate unless a number of clearly definable symptoms are present. For our purposes, we should substitute the terms, "heart burn" and "indigestion," since it is the discomfort that usually accompanies these simpler complications that is so often confused when one attempts the chancy game of self-diagnosis and self-medication.

Some disabling and killing diseases whose symptoms are often confused with indigestion and heart burn are pancreatitis, angina (as we have seen), gallstones, esophagitis, hiatus hernia (once a "fashionable" diagnosis) and a coronary or pulmonary thrombus or embolus. These latter conditions are generally called *infarctions*, a sudden occlusion in an organ caused by an obstruction of the circulation.

The sufferer from one of these potential killers is not always given as much advance warning as our unfortunate friend. But generally any persistent pain in the lower chest or upper gut that seems to respond to an antacid or a sedative, but recurs persistently, should be checked by a physician, and with no undue delay.

Fortunately the greatest number of problems are caused by the "I can't believe I ate the whole thing" syndrome, gorging ourselves until we balloon our diaphragms against the heart and lungs and get that "stuffy" feeling.

The clear implication in such commercial advertising is that one may "indulge" safely if he or she only has the foresight to have a bottle or tablet of the remedy at hand. However amusing it may be to watch a porcine actor grunt in discomfort until he has found relief, most physicians are far more pleased by the conservatism implied in an equally amusing commercial in which the man's abused stomach promises to meet him half way. ("I'll try if you will.")

In a small neighborhood drugstore, we counted sixty-three antacid preparations on shelves and in display boxes at the cash counter. (The druggist estimated that over 250 are available.) In 1972 OTC antacid sales amounted to $110 million. As of this writing final figures for 1973 were not available, but it was estimated that advertising budgets for antacids would total close to $45 million. In 1971, according to *Product Management Magazine,* ad budgets totalled $42.5 million. So it is no penny ante thing, this game being played by the OTC "gas house gang." And what the numbers indicate is alarming, for it means that millions of us *each day* are dosing ourselves for indigestion or sour stomach or other discomforts of the gastrointestinal system and in doing so are running the same risks as when we indulge in the self-diagnosis and prescription of analgesics, the headache and pain remedies discussed in Chapter 2.

It has been stated several times in these pages, and often in medical literature and in the general press, that OTC drugs have a perfectly legitimate place in our medicine cabinets and nightstand drawers—if they are used judiciously on small correctly self-diagnosed ailments and discomforts.

Again, it is obviously impractical to go running to the doctor for every little pain or discomfort, particularly when there is some very logical explanation for it, such as temporary distress from overeating or overdrinking.

The trouble lies in the fact that these small excesses are often committed habitually. We tend to live with these weekly hangovers as part of the price we pay for our self-indulgent lifestyle. And so we are prone to accept the recurring heart burn or headache or some other discomfort as "just another penalty for having a little fun." And time goes on and a disease, if it has taken hold, progresses, imitating the "harmless symptoms" until, finally, we are aware that something is wrong, go see the doctor and get the bad news.

Often we get into innocent trouble because we tend to believe the sponsor's advertising, or his labels. Because this is true, on Wednesday, April 4, 1973, the Food and Drug Administration issued a report that, for the time being, is really a "recommendation."

The recommendation, in effect, asks for a ban on nine antacid preparations. However, to those who do indulge in judicious self-medication, it came as a relief to find a number of the "old familiars" had been given a clean bill of health in so far as they were judged "safe and potentially effective" when used as directed for the specific disorders they were compounded to help.

Among them were such familiar dinnertime TV and radio commercial sponsors as the makers of Alka-Seltzer, Bromo-Seltzer, Rolaids, Tums, Gelusil and a clutch of milk of magnesia products.

Some qualifications were imposed, even on the best known brands. Particularly, the recommendation suggested that Alka-Seltzer, Bromo-Seltzer and other preparations that combine aspirin or some other analgesic with antacid ingredients would do better to specify on their labels that they should be used only for the relief of headache and indigestion. What the FDA wants in this regard is to avoid any implied suggestion that such preparations may also be useful in the self-administered treatment of gastric ulcers or other more serious disorders. The leading brands make no such claims.

There are, however, a great number of general claims that appear on OTC antacid remedies from time to time—allusions to the patent medicine's usefulness in relieving "nervous tension headaches," the "symptoms of the common cold" and others. The FDA discourages such claims unless unprejudiced tests prove that the claims have substance.

A few antacid products pretend some laxative properties. The FDA is determined that such claims may not be made on labels and in advertising if the laxative ingredient has been added to the antacid preparation to counter the constipating effect of one or more of the antacid ingredients.

In the April 4, 1973, report—really a *pro tempore* recommendation since an official regulation covering these products will not be issued for some months—the FDA took a skeptical look at an ingredient, a "de-gasser" known as simethicone.

It is used in several widely advertised products. There is no evidence the authors could find that there are any deleterious effects from the judicious use of antacid-anti-gas remedies that include it. But the FDA wants more reassurance. Accordingly, products including simethicone in their formulae will be given up to two years to prove their claims that the ingredient, in combination with the others in their remedies, actually does "cure upset stomach."

Doctor Murray Hoffstein makes a point to remind his patients that while a certain amount of self-medication is desirable, even necessary, the person who habitually takes a combination antacid and analgesic for an upset stomach may well run the risk of actually creating an ulcer where none existed. Moreover, if a peptic ulcer does exist, the ingestion of the analgesic quite probably will aggravate the condition.

"The aspirin or other analgesic may actually bring about serious pathological changes in an ulcer," warned Dr. Hoffstein. Some indication of how complicated proper diagnosis can be is gained from Dr. Hoffstein's observations to the authors about referred pain.

"Abdominal pain is not uncommon in pneumonia. Often it is due to referred pain or associated mesenteric *adenitis;* * it is very important to be checked for a chest ailment." The male half of this collaboration knows from bitter personal experience how devious these symptoms can be. At the risk of inflicting an "organ recital" upon the reader, it should be recounted briefly.

For no apparent reason, a severe and persistent pain occurred in the left ear. At first it was thought to be the result of a little injudicious snorkeling and skin diving in Hawaii. But it would not go away. A specialist looked at the ear and said there was some inflammation "trapped" behind the ear drum. There followed not one but two excruciating sessions in which the ear drum was pierced (without an anesthetic) and a tiny plastic drain tube was inserted. After the first inspection, the physician frowned and said quietly, "That's funny. There should be some discharge through the tube. Let's try again."

After three weeks of "trying again" the author said, "To hell with it!" and went to his general practitioner. Following a careful recounting of the weeks preceding the Hawaiian vacation—and a review of the medical history—the physician began to suspect referred pain.

*Inflammation of one or more lymph nodes.

X-rays were taken of the upper gastrointestinal tract where some inflammation was found. Tests indicated nothing more serious than "too much vacation," resulting in a slightly aggravated esophogus and congenital hiatus hernia. A few weeks of "easy on the sauce" and the mysterious ear ache disappeared. It seldom recurs. But when it does, a day or two of bland diet and no alcohol suffices and it goes away—without puncturing anything more serious than some easily deferred party plans. Rest and moderate eating does the trick with no medication.

But the devious referred pain in the ear, before it was finally identified for what it was, cost several hundred dollars in physicians' fees and laboratory work. It might very well have led to far more serious surgery. As to the congenital hiatus hernia which means that a "bit of the upper stomach is pressed upward into the opening in the diaphragm," Dr. Hoffstein says, "It is not uncommon and usually it is not serious."

Doctor Walter C. Alvarez has long maintained that there is too much fuss about hiatus herniation: "We feel that perhaps as many as a third of our men and women were born with the little space around the gullet and they never have any trouble with it."

Another harmless phenomenon that often frightens people into self-medication occurs as a result of being an unconscious "air swallower."

Not long ago, a member of the family, obviously in considerable emotional and physical distress, said, "I've had this pain in my upper abdomen—here. (She pointed to the usual area just below the breast bone.) So I went to the doctor and he had X-rays taken and I've got a very suspicious shadow under my heart."

Before long other doctors were called for consultation; among them a "chest man," a surgeon who specializes in operations involving the chest cavity. More X-rays were taken from every conceivable angle. Finally, after several months of tests, the anxious member of our family was told that it would be necessary to do an exploratory operation to make certain that the shadow was not "some malignancy." "We had better be certain," she was told.

Concerned, one of us suggested another opinion from a general practitioner in whom we have great confidence. The first thing he did was look at the X-rays. By now they covered a period of nearly five months.

After a very thoughtful examination of the pictures—with a radiologist he had much confidence in—it was determined that the "thing," whatever it was, had not changed in size. "If it were a malignancy that has appeared since your earlier X-rays during last year's physical examination, it would probably show signs of rapid growth—certainly some change in size—by now," the doctor concluded. And there had been no change except that in the latest pictures the crescent shaped shadow seemed to have flattened a bit at the top.

The decision to do the exploratory operation was postponed, much to the annoyance of the other physicians and surgeons who displayed circumspect professional anxiety.

During a series of office visits with the general practitioner, the member of the family confessed that she had been under great emotional stress due to the loss of her husband in an automobile accident and the necessity for reorganizing her life and taking care of a teenage daughter about to enter college.

Just prior to the X-rays that showed the mystery shadow, she had decided to take a difficult civil service examination. Her first try had failed by a fractional margin and she was preparing to retake it. All of this was going on at the time she first began feeling a little queasy.

The general practitioner suggested a mild sedative and a very simple diet until the pressure of the examination was over. The examination was passed and the widow in question suddenly found herself settling into a new career with the promise of job and retirement security. The daughter qualified for entrance to the university and suddenly the world was a brighter place.

The mysterious shadow was nothing more than an air bubble (distention)—swallowed air gulped down and trapped in the upper stomach during meals hastily eaten while tense. Subsequent X-rays show a normal conformation of the entire upper gastrointestinal area.

The potential-surgical candidate still shudders at the thought of what she might have gone through, "for nothing."

The point is, it would not have been for "nothing." It would have been for several thousands of dollars she did not have and for weeks of recuperation that might well have found her spending the rest of her years weakened from unnecessary surgery.

We do not imply that there was anything deliberately unethical in the faulty diagnosis of the "specialists." Many an honest mistake has been made by the most skilled professionals. But it is the patient who pays for those mistakes—often with his or her life.

So the possibilities for making mistakes not only lie in the area of self-diagnosis and medication. It is also possible for a highly trained physician to mistake the symptoms. In the case of the family member, the discomfort she felt was the manifestation of a superficial condition that quite probably would have been relieved if not "cured" by well-chosen OTC remedies. Taking the "proper precautions" in her case almost resulted in needless surgery. But as we have seen, the reverse is often true—self-diagnosis of "gastritis" and self-medication may result in masking symptoms of a potentially deadly disease.

The whole question, regardless of the part of the body involved, nets down to the employment of the *commonest* of common sense. One of the first things a person must be able to do to bring that sort of self-judgment into operation is to be absolutely certain that all of the pertinent facts are disclosed to self or to physician.

Unless the physician is a close relative who keeps tabs on the family, he has no way of knowing that you are being forgetful when you say, "Yes, I take an occasional drink but...."

An occasional drink may mean one or two a week to him. To you it may mean a double martini every night before dinner—and perhaps a highball later. For example, in many segments of our high pressure society, such a drink pattern might be considered "occasional" by the three-martinis-for-lunch set; whereas the physician might call it an habitual drinking pattern and look to the prolonged intake of alcohol as the gastrointestinal offender. In all the research and interviews the authors did not find a single doctor who regarded the regular though moderate use of alcohol as an "unimportant" factor diagnosing upper gastrointestinal disorders.

A realistic appraisal of personal habits, of job or career pressures, of marital climate, of any physical or emotional stress that may react on the physical machine—is absolutely essential in determining whether or not the "discomfort" in the gut or chest can be relieved safely by some OTC preparation. It is a tricky business—outwitting the "gas house gang."

11 The Vitamaniacs

If a little is good for you, it does not necessarily follow that more is better. Certainly nobody argues contrarily where unpleasant medications are concerned. But vitamins have a very special appeal to us.

First of all the word itself, *vitamin,* with the clear implication that it is a "vital" or a "life-giving" substance starts the subliminal process that has turned us into a generation of "vitamaniacs."

Antedeluvian tennis pro, Bobby Riggs, eats vitamin pills and capsules by the gross to stay the hand of Father Time. Billie Jean King is said to have taken them to stay the hand of Bobby Riggs. On talk shows, a score of movie and TV stars proudly boast of the magic combinations of vitamins that ensure everything from high ratings to hyperactive sex lives.

Supermarkets, super drug stores, health food stores and a number of combination rural gasoline station–country stores display shelves of vitamin pills that run the gamut from A to P. Mail order houses flood us with special offers, and dozens of nocturnal talk shows carry vitamin pill commercials that imply the "highly personal" endorsement of the amiable host who assures the listeners that he and his family cannot exist safely without them.

The irony of all this is simply that Americans who have the best overall diet of any country in the world, and therefore the least need for diet supplements, are the world's greatest overusers of vitamin pills.

One store in Los Angeles, "Vitamin Quota," says it sells *over one million pills and capsules each week.*

The 1972 "Statistical Abstract of the United States," issued by the Department of Commerce, placed vitamin production in 1970 at almost *23 million pounds.* That is more than 11,000 *tons!* Broken down into pills and capsules, the unit figure climbs into the *trillions.* Somebody with a bent for unusual arithmetic figured out that a vitamin pill is "dropped" down a gullet once every 0.214 second. That is pretty close to perpetual motion!

On the question of the need for supplementary vitamins in the average American diet, the proponents and the opponents face each other in about equal numbers. Also, the academic qualifications they display to support their various contentions are equally impressive.

Two distinguished Canadian heart specialists, Drs. Wilfred and Evan Shute, are convinced the work they have done shows that vitamin E plays an important role in the prevention of heart disease. But Dr. Campbell Moses of the American Heart Association is reported as being "unconvinced" that vitamin E has any appreciable effect on heart disease. Also, the food and nutrition board of the National Academy of Sciences-Natural Research Council (of which, world renowned nutritionist, Jean Mayer is a member) issued an announcement that extensive tests have failed to demonstrate therapeutic benefit from supplemental vitamin E.

Nobel chemist, Dr. Linus Pauling, is convinced that massive doses of vitamin C will both ward off or aid in curing the common cold. Doctor Edgar S. Gordon, Professor of Medicine at the University of Wisconsin, contends that the amounts of the various vitamins needed by normal animals or humans is very small and never exceeds a few micrograms to a few milligrams a day. "All available evidence," says Dr. Gordon, "indicates that excessive quantities supplied through the diet or administered artificially are lost through renal excretion."

The number of medical doctors who feel that most of us get all the vitamins and minerals we need in our daily diets is legion. Most of these physicians will also acknowledge that in certain instances, where some physiological aberration is found that affects the utilization of one or more of the essential vitamins, it may be necessary to add them as a supplement.

The appeal of the *miracle cure promise* is enormous. It is almost impossible to shake the faith of a true vitamin believer. Their conviction is no less than that of the pilgrims who carry their infirmities to the Shrine of Our Lady of Fatima or to Lourdes.

"If I *think* I feel better, I *feel* better!" said one young man who was into health foods and vitamins. No metaphysician and perhaps few "just plain" physicians would dispute that, insofar as it goes. In carefully controlled tests, *placebos* have been known to effect some remarkable cures too. And it all took place "between the ears."

Doctor Edward Shanbrom, Associate Clinical Professor of Medicine and Pathology at the U.C.L.A. School of Medicine in Westwood, an internationally recognized hematologist whose research work has been carried on in many parts of the world, including regions in Africa inhabited by primitive tribes, takes issue with those responsible for the removal of folic acid from the B complex vitamins. He feels that while many of us take vitamins we do not need, it is possible for us to be deficient in one or more vitamins that are necessary to good nutrition.

"Folic acid deficiency is the second most common nutritional deficiency in the world," Dr. Shanbrom said. Iron is the first!

"A pregnant woman will become folic-acid deficient in her third trimester. Moreover, folic acid deficiency may be increased by the drugs she takes. Many drugs become antagonistic to folic acid."

Under further questioning about sources of folic acid, Dr. Shanbrom said, "It is found principally in liver and in leafy green vegetables. It can also be synthesized. The trouble is, folic acid is a fragile substance and cooking destroys it. It takes only three minutes of boiling to destroy it completely."

When asked why the FDA ordered folic acid removed from most B complex formulae, he said, "too much folic acid may mask pernicious anemia symptoms. But this is not a widespread disease now. When it is diagnosed, vitamin B_{12} can be given. Pernicious anemia patients have an absorption problem. But it is a relative one. If massive doses of B_{12} are given, the patient will absorb sufficient amounts. B_{12}, by the way, is one of the cheapest vitamins to produce."

Folic acid is available in special pregnancy capsules but in Dr. Shanbrom's opinion the quantities are far too small.

"A normal person needs about one milligram a day. But a pregnant woman may need from five to ten milligrams daily. In that event, she must get special folic acid capsules—under the direction of her physician, of course."

Contrary to the opinion held by some, Dr. Shanbrom also feels that because lack of iron is our number one deficiency, even here in the United States, the FDA is correct in following the advice of its scientists to increase the amount of iron in breads.

In the old days when we cooked in iron pots and drank well water containing rust in the pump pipes and when we had cast iron water mains, we got vital amounts of iron in our diets. But the principal source came from the whole grains and the unprocessed flour we used in baking breads. Shortly before World War I, new milling processes that produced bleached white flour took many nutritious elements, including iron, from the grains.

Doctor Shanbrom feels that even in our relatively affluent society we may be deficient in iron by serious amounts. In his opinion, the amounts of iron to be added will pose little if any risk. "Women, especially," he pointed out, "lose significant amounts of iron during menstruation. Then they take aspirin to cope with the cramps and it, in turn, causes more blood loss." He does not regard as serious the possibility that additional iron will result in male sterility or in liver damage. Many of those consulted agreed that since we are not a great bread-eating nation the risk of getting toxic amounts of iron from that source is negligible, even though iron is also added to some of our dry cereals.

It is fruitless to spend pages setting down the various arguments and displaying the results of the tests, controlled and otherwise, on which these disparate conclusions have been reached.

In fairness, it should be pointed out that the skeptics do not contend that vitamins are of no use. They simply say, and it may be a debatable contention, that those Americans who avail themselves of a reasonably varied food supply including meat, cereals, fruits *(especially citrus)*, vegetables and dairy products and use care in the preparation are getting all the vitamins and minerals necessary to maintain excellent health. Of course, this assumes a normally functioning physical machine to start with.

Because citrus fruits are one of the principal natural sources of many basic nutritional elements, when Dr. Linus Pauling first propounded his theory that mega-doses of vitamin C (ascorbic acid) could prevent and aid in the curing of the common cold, the citrus industry, feeling it might have an exciting merchandising "hook," looked into the tests being done in a number of places.

"It would have been a tremendous boon to us to help Dr. Pauling prove his theory," said Don Heller, Assistant Vice President, Marketing Services, for Sunkist Growers, "but we were unable to find any supporting clinical evidence of a convincing nature (to Sunkist's scientists) that the theory would prove out."

It would take roughly one thousand oranges to provide the mega-doses of ascorbic acid that Dr. Pauling advocates, if that superior citrus fruit were the only source. But certainly, for normal amounts of vitamin C, important amounts of vitamins A and B complex and appreciable amounts of important minerals, including potassium, the orange may be one of the world's finest health foods.

In the course of researching this chapter, the authors read several hundred papers and articles representing all aspects of the vitamin controversy. There can be no question that the proponents and opponents of vitamin therapy are sincere and well qualified men and women. But the dominant fact that strikes an investigative reporter is the apparent lack of in-depth nutritional knowledge by the so-called general practitioner.

A number of physicians confessed that while they had studied basic nutrition in medical school, their practices now left too little time to stay abreast of new material. Moreover, a number of physicians candidly admitted that much of the basics they had learned years ago had "dimmed" a bit. "We tend to rely too much on data provided by pharmaceutical houses in support of their products. Their research is often good; but it may be biased too. We should make time to do more reading," said one distinguished physician who facetiously describes himself as a "gutologist." He went on to say that he is making time now to investigate some very interesting work being done by Dr. Willard Visek, Professor of Animal Science at Cornell University:

> Doctor Visek has produced some convincing evidence that the high incidence of bowel cancer in this country, and I see much too much of it in my patients, may be caused by ingesting too much protein in our diets. The Visek studies seem to show a definite correlation between the incidence of bowel cancer and the amount of protein consumed by members of some societies. In countries with high protein intake, there appears to be more such cancer. In our own affluent society, this becomes a critical nutritional problem.

If physicians themselves are remiss, then certainly so are we, their patients, for not taking advantage of the excellent popular literature available. The *Reader's Digest,* "I Am Joe's——" and "I Am Jane's——," series makes excellent elementary reading. The articles describe in the clearest, most interesting language, the functioning of our basic organs. Without developing a morbid preoccupation with its functions, it is hard to think of anything that should interest us more than the physiological machine that takes us through this life experience.

In the process of informing themselves for this work, the authors had the good fortune to come across a small softcover edition published by the University of Chicago Press' *Phoenix Science Series.* It is titled *Food for Life,* edited by our friend and consultant, Dr. Ralph W. Gerard, one of the world's most distinguished physiologists and Dean Emeritus of Biological Sciences at the University of California, Irvine, and first Dean of the University's Graduate Division.

Subtitled, "A readable survey of the essentials of nutrition," the book contains contributions by such authorities as Richard J. Block, Norman Jolliffe, Clive M. McCay, Sedgwick E. Smith and Samuel Soskin. The material has been skillfully brought together by Dr. Gerard in a most "readable" manner and a trip through its pages is a fascinating adventure. After taking this trip, one can hardly take for granted the human body and its miraculous mechanisms for converting food and drink into body building blocks and energy.

Doctor Murray Hoffstein at New York's Mt. Sinai Hospital underlined the need for more nutritional knowledge. "We come out of medical school knowing a great deal about basic nutritional needs, but if our primary objective is health maintenance rather than the treatment of disease, then we should know a great deal more about the interaction of the nutritional elements in the foods we eat." Many medical doctors had gone "back to school" to add to and refine their knowledge.

New research techniques are revealing much more about the complicated relationships of the chemical components of the human body and the infinitely delicate mechanisms that keep them harmonized. Even those doctors who were skeptical of the "miracle uses" of vitamins C, B^6 and E displayed no symptoms of a closed mind. All were willing to concede that future research might well confirm some of the claims now being made. But, as scientists, they could not abandom themselves to the sudden enthusiasm for new things displayed by some of their colleagues, particularly when there seemed to be as much negative as positive evidence. For instance, clinical histories are filled with cases of vitamin A toxicity. Much damage has been done to the kidneys and liver from self-prescribed overdoses of vitamin A. While it is true that in most cases the patients improved when the vitamin was withdrawn, doctors acknowledge the possibility of residual damage.

"Once the physical machine has suffered that sort of damage it simply is not as good as it was before the damage was sustained," they say.

Doctor Robert E. Hodges, Professor of Internal Medicine at the University of California at Davis, and Chief of the Nutritional Section, speaking at a Stanford University conference in August 1973, at which Dr. Pauling "plumped" for his theory, reported on a test conducted by Russian doctors nine years earlier. The results of these tests showed sixteen of twenty pregnant women who were given six grams of vitamin C daily suffered abortions.

Doctor Hodges also presented evidence that large amounts of vitamin C may cause kidney stones. Speaking to Dr. Pauling's contention, Dr. Hodges concluded by saying, "I wouldn't advise taking vitamin C. There is no real evidence that it prevents colds. It may relieve symptoms, but you can do that with other medication such as aspirin."

The health food advocates immediately countered with their favorite argument: "If both relieve the symptoms, then why not use the one that can't hurt you, vitamin C?"

The unrestricted use of vitamin A has been identified as the cause of another serious ailment, one whose symptoms have led to unnecessary and very dangerous operations.

Patients who have overdosed themselves with vitamin A have complained of pressure inside the skull. Some of these persons have described the sensation as "a feeling like something is growing inside of my head and making pressure. It is driving me crazy. I feel like I want to make a hole in my skull and let the pressure out."

Statements such as that have led physicians to suspect brain tumor. In an effort to make a positive diagnosis, the patient has been subjected to a costly course of encephalograms. When the X-rays reveal nothing, but the symptoms persist and grow more acute, there is a very real danger that the physician, unaware that the patient has been overdosing with vitamin A, may feel he has no recourse but to operate and do some exploring. It hardly needs to be said that there are few more dangerous places in the human body to conduct surgical exploration.

As the possible side effects of vitamin overdosing are better known, most physicians are questioning patients more persistently, conducting in-depth verbal cross-examinations in an effort to elicit information the patient may have forgotten or is withholding.

In one of his novels, *Condition Pink,* the male half of this collaboration had a college professor character admit that "it is possible to be logical without being correct." That line was adopted as a slogan by his daughter's class at the University of Denver and was displayed in a large banner in the dorm. The point was that perfectly logical conclusions can be drawn from incomplete evidence, and the authors could find no authority who would categorically state that all the evidence is now available in the whole complicated nutritional inquiry.

If one wants to predict what is likely to happen tomorrow, the best thing to do is study what happened yesterday. There are recurring patterns in human behavior and in accomplishment. One of the brightest threads in the pattern is man's aspiration to better his lot.

No census exists as to the number of experiments in vitamin therapy that are presently on-going. Everyone interviewed agreed they must run into the tens of thousands, worldwide. No one doubts for an instant that out of this work will come some dramatic breakthroughs and that these new discoveries, when they come, will disprove some popular theories and prove some presently unpopular ones.

All the contentions on the part of the health food fadists that we should take vitamin supplements because our modern refined foods have been robbed of much of their nourishment, despite the fact that vitamins and minerals are added, seem somehow unreasonable in the face of the professional nutritionists' contention that in this country nobody need suffer from an inadequate diet. All the basic foods we need are available, everywhere in the land. Those who are not getting proper nourishment are suffering from poor eating habits, not lack of available good food.

Survey after survey of the eating habits of people in various regions of the country confirm this as a fact. Dietary deficiencies in the South and in the Southwest are the result of faulty eating patterns established several generations ago. It is true that in the beginning such patterns may well have represented the best the underprivileged could obtain at the time. But modern food processing and transportation and distribution have changed all that.

In scores of small country stores visited in all parts of the United States and Mexico, the authors did not find a single one in which any one of the four basic food groups was not available. (Several leading nutritionists, among them, Harvard's Dr. Jean Mayer, say the basic four food groups is an oversimplification and should be expanded to the W.W. II basic *seven,* since some foods rightfully belong in categories of their own.)

Moreover, in the South where the dietary deficiencies are said to be most prevalent, the authors found the lowest food prices in the nation. This was not the first but the second time we have researched basic food prices within an eighteen month period.* What emerges is clear evidence that if a family—even one on food stamps—wishes to include all the basic nutrients in its daily diet, they can do so. "Trouble is," said one storekeeper near Greenville, Mississippi, "a lot of folks just feel more comfortable with blackeyed peas, sidemeat and pan bread." In that same little store, a lot of money went for soft drinks, candy and other sweets. Physicians admitted there was a troublesome incidence of undernourishment in the area.

Among the young people, various local and state agencies try to compensate for lack of minerals and vitamins with good school lunch programs. They are finding that proper nutrition is one of the hardest subjects to teach in schools.

*See Cooley, *How To Avoid the Retirement Trap,* Nash, 1972; Popular Library, 1973.

What is done in the classroom is too often undone at home through ignorance or indifference.

It is largely because of this that the proponents of vitamin supplement programs fight so hard for their point of view. Their position was stated with some eloquence by a school district nutritionist in Louisiana:

> It's heartbreaking to see these young children growing up with deficient physical machines when a few simple changes in their diets could change their whole physical and mental potential. It is the parents we must change and the indifference we encounter makes us want to scream out loud against their stupidity.

Because of the potential danger of overdosing with vitamins, the Food and Drug Administration on August 1, 1973, banned the nonprescription sale of vitamins A and D in high concentrations because it has been established that they are "clearly dangerous" in large quantities.

The regulation, which took effect sixty days after the issuance, requires the buyer to provide the druggist with a doctor's prescription for doses over 10,000 International Units of vitamin A and about 400 IUs of vitamin D.

The limit of vitamin D is the same as the RDA—the *recommended daily allowance*. The limit on vitamin A is somewhat higher than the RDA.

In addition to the pressure in the skull that mimics brain tumor, the FDA revealed that large doses of both vitamins over a period of time may retard the growth of children.

More restrictions are coming, particularly on vitamins combined with other substances that have no recognized scientific value in nutrition and on vitamin and food supplements containing more than three times the recommended daily allowance of any one vitamin.

However constructive these new safeguards may be, the flaw is obvious: no regulation, as now written, can keep a customer from buying vitamins A and D in *smaller* International Unit capsules and pills and simply taking more of them. The result will be the same—dangerous overdosing. Nobody in Washington, D.C., was optimistic about the possibility that the public would heed the warning. The dilemma, of course, lies in the fact that the only way we can be protected against our own damn foolishness is to put all these items on the restricted list. That is patently impossible. "We must rely on long-term public education," said one FDA official. "That is definitely the 'hard way'; but it's the only way we can accomplish our aims without throwing the whole health care establishment into chaos."

How long ago did this vitamin controversy begin? For all practical purposes, it started in 1911 with the discovery of vitamin B_1 by the Polish biochemist, Casimir Funk. In that year, Dr. Funk isolated a substance in unpolished rice that prevented the dietary deficiency disease called beriberi. The word "vitamin" is generally credited to the Polish biochemist who combined "vita," the Latin word for "life," with the chemical term "amine."

In time, due to the work of such pioneers as Funk, Goldberger, Wheeler, Elvehjen, Williams, Szent-Gyorgi and others, a whole family of vitamins was discovered. In the process, a great deal of new information about the nature of our physiological machines came to light. As far back as 1867, niacin, then called nicotinic acid, had been derived from nicotine. It was used in the treatment of "black tongue" in dogs and later was used in the treatment of pellagra in humans—a closely related deficiency disease.

As time went by, more was learned about the nature of these mysterious substances that seemed to have miraculous powers to rid man of some of his most persistent ailments.

It came to be understood that vitamins differed widely in composition and that there are two classes: the fat solubles A, D, E and K; and the water solubles B complex and C.

Although some thirty different vitamins have been isolated and named, fewer than a dozen have been studied sufficiently to have been designated as "essential" by the Board of the National Academy of Sciences, National Research Council. They are:

Vitamin A is an essential fat-soluble vitamin needed for vision as it is a part of the purple visual pigment, rhodopsin. It is necessary for the maintenance of the thin layer of cells (the epithelium) which lines the trachea (wind pipe), conjunctiva (eyeball linings), hair follicles and the kidneys. It is also important for good bone growth.

Butter, cream, egg yoke and liver contain vitamin A; as do the many green and yellow vegetables which convert carotene into vitamin A in the intestinal lining.

It is an easily stored and slowly excreted vitamin; therefore, repeated doses may lead to accumulation and "poisoning"—anemia, enlarged liver, headaches, changes in bones and hair, low-grade fever and weight loss.

The daily recommended allowance varies from as much as 6,000 IU for nursing mothers to as few as 1,400 IU for infants. (See the Food and Nutrition Board's chart on daily allowances for individual variations.)

Vitamin B_1 (thiamine, aneurin) is an important water soluble vitamin for optimum function of the nervous system and the heart. Best sources for thiamine are found in most meats, poultry, milk, eggs, peanut butter, wheat germ, whole grain, enriched breads and cereals and brewer's yeast. As with most vitamins in the B category, you will find the recommended daily allowance is between 1 and 2 milligrams. Folacin (400 mg) and B_{12} (3mg) are the exceptions.

Vitamin B_2 (riboflavin) maintains the tone of the mucous membrane and skin and is essential for proper growth ahd tissue function. Recommended daily allowance is between 1 and 2 milligrams. Although widely distributed in foods, it is destroyed on exposure to light.

Vitamin B_6 (pyridoxine) functions in the metabolizing or processing of amino acids, the basic component of protein. It is useful in preventing cavities in children. It relieves a form of neuritis and is particularly beneficial during pregnancies. Again, the recommended daily allowance is between 1 and 2 milligrams per day.

Vitamin B_{12} (cobalamin) is one of the most biologically active substances known. It is vital for the normal development of red blood cells. If treated early by a physician, *pernicious anemia* (patients lack a substance in gastric juices and cannot absorb vitamin B_{12} in food) is no longer the fatal disease it once was due to the discovery of B_{12}.

Vitamin B complex consists of thiamine, B_1; riboflavin, B_2; niacin, pyridoxine, B_6; and panthothenic acid; together with the "anti-anemia" vitamins; (folic acid)* and vitamin B_{12}. To this list may be added choline that is said to prevent fat deposits from building up in the liver, biotin which is necessary for the production of essential fatty substances and pantothenic acid which we need for the metabolism of carbohydrates.

Deficiency in the B complex is most often brought on by abnormal circumstances: circulatory diseases, leukemia, fever, hyperthyroidism, diarrhea or inflammation of the digestive tract. (The administration of oral antibiotics has an effect on the utilization of the B complex.) Then, too, the body may use the vitamins abnormally in such diseases as cirrhosis of the liver and diabetes mellitus.

Vitamin C (ascorbic acid) is a water-soluble substance essential for the circulatory system, healthy connective tissue, bones and teeth. It is also necessary to the body's handling of iron. And it plays an important role in the function of the adrenal gland. It is particularly useful in stressful conditions such as burns and extensive injuries. We have known for some time that without the C vitamin during infancy, serious illnesses may develop. Now we know this also applies to the elderly too, particularly to those who live alone and have poor eating habits. And, of course, we're all familiar with that disease, scurvy.

Citrus fruits, tomatoes, cabbage and potatoes are the main sources of vitamin C. But exposure to heat or light easily diminishes its potency.

Check the table in this section for recommended daily requirements which can vary from 35 milligrams for in-

---

*Folic acid (Folacin) has been deleted because it can mask the symptoms of pernicious anemia. There is controversy on this deletion. Many doctors say that there are too many people with a folacin deficiency.

fants to 60 milligrams for male adults. Taken in recommended doses, vitamin C is basically nontoxic.

Vitamin D is a fat-soluble food substance essential to the calcium and phosphorus content of body fluids: it is part of a group of related substances chemically resembling cholesterol and certain hormones.

This "sunshine vitamin" is unique because the body is only partially dependent on food sources due to the formation of the vitamin in the skin upon exposure to sunlight. Today, vitamin D enriched milk, margarine and fatty fish along with exposure to the sun meets most requirements in healthy individuals. We seldom see rickets in the United States anymore; but if more vitamin D is needed for prevention of this disease, follow the doctor's prescribed dose very closely, especially for infants.

The recommended daily allowance for healthy individuals is 400 IU or 10 milligrams of crystalline vitamin D_2 (calciferol) for light skinned races. Dark pigmented people require about 50 percent more because of the pigment's interference with vitamin D production.

While an extremely important vitamin, *massive* doses may have serious toxic reactions: deposit of calcium in abnormal sites, elevation of serum calcium levels, vomiting, diarrhea and kidney failure that can be fatal.

Vitamin E (alpha-tocopherol) is another fat-soluble vitamin. We know it's essential because it seems to be a vital antioxidant. But there is still much to be learned about its role in metabolism. Meat, fish, poultry, eggs, wheat germ and vegetable oil among other foods contain vitamin E. However, the processing and storage of foods can result in a significant loss of the vitamin. One source said as much as 90 percent in some foods.

Vitamin E was found to prolong the life-span of experimental animals. It was also found that babies with an uncommon anemia were also deficient in vitamin E.

Again, check the table herein for the daily dietary allowance as it varies with one's age and sex.

Vitamin K (naphthoquinone), also a fat-soluble vitamin, is

RECOMMENDED DAILY DIETARY ALLOWANCE

Fat-soluble Vitam

	(years) from Up to	Wt. (lb)	Ht. (in)	Energy (kcal)	Protein (g)	Vita-min A Activity (IU)	Vita-min D (IU)	Vita-min Activ-ity (IU
INFANTS	0.0-0.5	14	24	kg × 117	kg × 2.2	1,400	400	4
	0.5-1.0	20	28	kg × 108	kg × 2.0	2,000	400	5
CHILDREN	1-3	28	34	1,300	23	2,000	400	7
	4-6	44	44	1,800	30	2,500	400	9
	7-10	66	54	2,400	36	3,300	400	10
MALES	11-14	97	63	2,800	44	5,000	400	12
	15-18	134	69	3,000	54	5,000	400	15
	19-22	147	69	3,000	52	5,000	400	15
	23-50	154	69	2,700	56	5,000		15
	51+	154	69	2,400	56	5,000		15
FEMALES	11-14	97	62	2,400	44	4,000	400	10
	15-18	119	65	2,100	48	4,000	400	11
	19-22	128	65	2,100	46	4,000	400	12
	23-50	128	65	2,000	46	4,000		12
	51+	128	65	1,800	46	4,000		12
PREGNANCY				+300	+30	5,000	400	15
LACTATION				+500	+20	6,000	400	15

[1] The allowances are intended to provide for individual variations among most normal persons as they live in the United States under usual environmental stresses. Diets should be based on a variety of common foods in order to provide other nutrients for which human requirements have been less well defined.

REVISED 1973

	Water-soluble Vitamins								Minerals			
Ascorbic Acid (mg)	Folacin (μg)²	Niacin (mg)	Riboflavin (mg)	Thiamin (mg)	Vitamin B6 (mg)	Vitamin B12 (μg)	Calcium (mg)	Phosphorus (mg)	Iodine (μg)	Iron (mg)	Magnesium (mg)	Zinc (mg)
35	50	5	0.4	0.3	0.3	0.3	360	240	35	10	60	3
35	50	8	0.6	0.5	0.4	0.3	540	400	45	15	70	5
40	100	9	0.8	0.7	0.6	1.0	800	800	60	15	150	10
40	200	12	1.1	0.9	0.9	1.5	800	800	80	10	200	10
40	300	16	1.2	1.2	1.2	2.0	800	800	110	10	250	10
45	400	18	1.5	1.4	1.6	3.0	1,200	1,200	130	18	350	15
45	400	20	1.8	1.5	1.8	3.0	1,200	1,200	150	18	400	15
45	400	20	1.8	1.5	2.0	3.0	800	800	140	10	350	15
45	400	18	1.6	1.4	2.0	3.0	800	800	130	10	350	15
45	400	16	1.5	1.2	2.0	3.0	800	800	110	10	350	15
45	400	16	1.3	1.2	1.6	3.0	1,200	1,200	115	18	300	15
45	400	14	1.4	1.1	2.0	3.0	1,200	1,200	115	18	300	15
45	400	14	1.4	1.1	2.0	3.0	800	800	100	18	300	15
45	400	13	1.2	1.0	2.0	3.0	800	800	100	18	300	15
45	400	12	1.1	1.0	2.0	3.0	800	800	80	10	300	15
60	800	+2	+0.3	+0.3	2.5	4.0	1,200	1,200	125	18+³	450	20
60	600	+4	+0.5	+0.3	2.5	4.0	1,200	1,200	150	18	450	25

² Microgram.
³ This increased requirement cannot be met by ordinary diets; therefore, the use of supplemental iron is recommended.

essential for normal function of the liver and as a blood coagulant. It is often used as a preoperative prophylaxis and it may be administered to the mother or the newborn infant to reduce the danger of hemorrhage. As you can see, this is not a vitamin to prescribe for oneself. Among the sources of vitamin K are, green vegetables, cabbage, cauliflower and *soybean* oil.

Interestingly enough, as recently as 1972, Dr. Armand J. Quick of the Medical College of Wisconsin, reported that he thought he had discovered a new vitamin. It is called Q. As the eminent developer of a widely used test for blood coagulation qualities, Dr. Quick's discovery that a *soybean* extract belonging to the phospholipid family hastens the clotting of blood in test tubes apparently has been confirmed by other researchers.

Although there are more than sixty nutrients (vitamins and minerals) recognized as essential in human nutrition, the RDA gives recommended amounts for only seventeen. Of these, you will note that only ten vitamins are included in the RDA.

The worst that one can say about the vitamin family is that it is a "mixed bag" of blessings. Nobody argues the basic contention that vitamins are vital to good health. But there is plenty of room for thoughtful discussion about the *"how many–how much–how long?"* aspect of the discussion. What it nets down to, really, is a question of wasted dollars and common sense.

If it is true—and there is much evidence that it may be— that most of the water soluble vitamins not needed by our bodies are excreted, then we are really "putting down the drain" a lot of money that could be better spent on nutritionally sound foods that benefit the entire physical machine. At the very least, we are wasting those units that represent an overdose.

The health food faddists have much reason on their side when they say that it is better to get the full spectrum of vitamin and minerals in "natural foods" since the possibility for overdosing is negligible.

"Nobody in his right mind is going to get too much carotene and vitamin A by eating five pounds of carrots at a sitting," said one former registered nurse who is the "mother superior" of a local health food store patronized by a hoard of enthusiastic young cultists.

And still, excesses are possible. We have seen this same delightful lady express the juice of two pounds of carrots in an electrical extractor, serve it up in a plastic container with a straw and watch while the eager young customer slurps it down to the last drop. "Sometimes he drinks three of those a day," she admitted.

Mentioned earlier were the numerous research projects underway whose purposes are a much broader, more definitive knowledge of the functions of vitamins in human nutrition.

While very little proved data have come from these investigations as yet, there is much interesting and some hopeful evidence that several vitamins, used under controlled conditions, may aid in preventing cancer, heart disease, diabetes, certain kidney disorders and a number of diseases of the gastrointestinal system. Most of the work is being done on laboratory animals.

Work on-going at the University of California, Los Angeles, and at the University of Hawaii, seems to indicate that one of the B vitamins, nicotinamide, can arrest cancer in rats. The vitamin is said to be present in normal cells but is not found in cancerous cells. The result was a slowing down or stopping of uncontrolled cell growth.

What these teams of scientists are hoping to prove is that nicotinamide will be useful in the prevention and treatment of cancer in humans. Those experiments have not yet begun.

In another series of experiments being conducted at Penn State, there is hopeful evidence that ascorbic acid, vitamin C, may be useful in removing cholesterol from the bloodstream. Experiments on rats have shown dramatic results. But there is a long experimental "row to hoe" before it can be proved that the same procedure will reduce cholesterol in the human vascular system and thereby reduce our susceptibility to heart attacks.

Both vitamins E and B_6 are being exhaustively researched as possible aids in preventing such apparently unrelated diseases as numbness of the hands and arms due to coronary thrombosis. Moreover, it is believed by many researchers that the aging process can be slowed down by introducing controlled amounts of vitamin E in the diet. This controversial vitamin appears to have the power to slow down the oxidation process, the burning up of cells, associated with aging. There is evidence that in our anxiety to cut down on saturated fats that speed up the production of cholesterol and increase the risk of atherosclerosis and arteriosclerosis that we are ingesting too much polyunsaturated fat. This type of fat has a tendency to oxidize more quickly in the body. Accordingly, biochemists feel that additional amounts of an antioxidant should be taken to stabilize the process. Many research scientists feel that vitamin E, and probably B_6 as well, will aid in the "slow down."

Most of the biochemists and physicians conducting these experiments agree that the interrelation of the whole vitamin family is a subtle, infinitely complicated phenomenon, that no single vitamin, without the presence of at least some of the others, has the potential of affecting a "miracle cure" of any of the stubborn diseases that thus far have eluded the scientists.

Of the vitamins needed for proper physiological functioning, vitamin D is the only one that can be produced in the body. This so-called "sunshine vitamin" is essential for the young and old alike since it helps to maintain the proper calcium and phosphate balance necessary for the condition physicians call "skeletal integrity."

That is "lab jarg" for healthy bone structure. To repeat, vitamin D is formed in our skin when we subject it to sunlight. Most children and adults who spend at least a part of each week in the sun run little risk of being deficient in vitamin D. In the unlikely event that we should be deficient, we receive adequate amounts of supplementary vitamin D in the fortified milk we drink.

When all the pros and cons are reduced to a common sense denominator, the scientific consensus may be simply stated: if you are eating a good variety of foods in the basic categories, meats, cereals, fruits and vegetables and dairy products, there is little likelihood that you need any supplementary vitamins to maintain optimum health.

If, on the other hand, your diet contains a reasonable variety of these foods and something still appears to be wrong, the place to go is to your physician. If he cannot deduce from your history and further questioning what the trouble is, he will order a series of tests that, in all likelihood, will reveal the trouble.

If it is a dietary deficiency because of an inability to absorb one or more of the critical vitamins, he may prescribe supplements in carefully monitored doses. These may be given by injection. The last place to go for diagnostic counsel is to one of the health food stores. Even if you are fortunate enough to find one that employs a graduate nutritionist, the task of identifying the problem by a correct reading of symptoms belongs to the physician.

As far as vitamin E is concerned, since there seems to be no danger of toxicity, and since most American diets are thought to be slightly deficient in the three tocopherols in vitamin E that function as antioxidants, there may be some general benefit in taking the 200 to 300 IUs daily that appear to be the amount needed to effectively control the metabolism of both saturated and polyunsaturated fats. We found a number of doctors who were taking vitamin E on that assumption.

As to the dire effects of our great national *vitamania*, they seem to be relatively few beyond those associated with the overdoses of vitamins A and D, which prompted the new FDA regulations on over-the-counter dispensing: the apparent danger to pregnant women in overdosing with vitamin C (this latter on the assumption that the Russian tests were significant) and to some individuals, one potentially very serious side effect involving folic acid, a constituent of vitamin B complex.

In the fall of 1971, the FDA ordered the amount of folic acid drastically reduced in multivitamin preparations when it was found that doses in excess of 0.1 milligram might mask a vitamin B_{12} deficiency while allowing certain neurological damage to progress in persons with pernicious anemia.

Until the studies alerted the FDA to this very grave danger, the usual dose of folic acid was 5 milligrams. Autopsies revealed that a number of deaths from pernicious anemia were almost certainly caused by the masking effect which concealed the vital B_{12} deficiency until too late.

Most of the OTC preparations simply removed folic acid from their B complex formulae and packed it in 0.1, 0.5 and 1 milligram tablets, the latter dosage being the limit set by the FDA.* If a physician runs tests and finds folic acid deficiency, he may prescribe therapeutic doses of *folinic* acid, a well-absorbed, orally administered reduced form of folic acid.

There is little question now that folic acid deficiency syndromes are common. If they are suspected, the physician has at his disposal a series of plasma (blood) tests that will indicate the level of concentration at which point the proper course of treatment will be prescribed. Even though it may be bought over-the-counter in the FDA approved strengths, folic acid is not a vitamin to be monkeyed with.

It is not uncommon to hear pregnant women counseling each other to take folic acid because it will aid in the development of the fetus during the gestation period and later is required for normal lactation. Actually, it has been established that a normal female requires only 0.3 milligram of folic acid during gestation, an amount easily received in a

---

*According to the revised 1973 RDA table, this recommendation has been changed to 400 *micrograms*.

well-balanced diet.* However, many physicians prescribe small supplementary doses. Otherwise a normal person needs no more than 0.05 milligrams (now increased to 400 micrograms).

Alcoholics are often advised—usually by other sufferers from the same disease—to take folic acid. There appears to be a sound clinical reason for treating acute alcoholism with folic acid, among other things. But under no circumstances should such treatment be undertaken on the advice of anyone other than a physician

Anticonvulsants given to epileptics also may create a folic acid deficiency that can result in anemia and a sense of mental confusion. A situation such as this requires the most skillful medical care since the administering of additional acid to balance out the deficiency may also result in modifying the anticonvulsant effect. It is a damned-if-you-do, damned-if-you-don't situation and self-diagnosis and self-treatment is the height of folly.

To go back to the original observation that because a little is good for you it does not necessarily follow that more is better, the only sensible course to follow where vitamins—or any other food or medicine that has the potential to "kill or cure"—are concerned is to spend the time and the money to get expert medical consultation before self-prescribing a course of over-the-counter drugs.

You may say, "I can't afford to go running to the doctor with every little thing." Very few people can; and certainly the doctor doesn't want to see you every time you "imagine" you are coming down with something.

But if you are eating a well-balanced diet, you are not hung up on excessive damaging habits such as smoking and drinking and you feel "poorly" over a considerable period of time, you should go to the doctor for a thorough physical checkup.

---

*Curiously enough, many scientists now feel that these "wives' tales" may be closer to the truth, witness the new recommended daily allowances

Chances are it will be nothing more serious than a deficiency or a superficial malfunction that, if caught in time, will respond easily. We have seen persons, particularly older people living on limited fixed incomes, spend hundreds of dollars on health food remedies and nostrums because they "couldn't afford to go to the doctor."* Such action makes neither fiscal nor physiological sense. In the end, the relatively few dollars spent on a physical exam would be a miniscule amount when compared with the cost of hospitalization and surgery—even with the dubious assistance of Medicare.

There is no substitute for a simple but varied diet. Everything most of us need to maintain a normal vitamin and mineral level in our bodies is available in any neighborhood market. True, food is not as cheap as it was. And neither are medical services. But given a choice—and we have one—there is little question of what the priority should be.

*Cooley, How To Avoid the Retirement Trap, Nash, 1972; and Popular Library, 1973.

12 Diet Pills, the Great "Take it off" Put-on

Despite all the reams of advertising, provocative claims and downright promises, the consensus of expert medical opinion of diet pills is very clear: *if you are overweight, remember that prescription drugs have not been shown to help over an extended period of time and may help you only a little over the short term.*

*Any decision to use them should take into account the fact that some drugs do cause drug dependence and have been widely abused.**

Most of the pills and capsules prescribed by doctors for obesity contain appetite suppressants. While scientists agree that the drugs seem to inhibit the appetite, they are not certain how this takes place.

But they are very certain these drugs, called *anoretics* in the medical profession, are potentially dangerous since most, but not all of them, contain *amphetamine* which we have seen to be a psychoactive, habit-forming drug.

Early in 1973, the FDA concluded an exhaustive review of anoretic drugs: anoretics have a very limited usefulness in the treatment of obesity and the essential ingredient, amphetamine ("pep pills" or "uppers") can send a persistent user of these reducing pills and capsules on a "bad trip." If one is not up on the drug culture lingo, a "bad trip" is a reaction resulting in bizarre, psychotic behavior and the subsequent torment of withdrawal.

The temptation to find some sort of a pill that will do the job that should be done by will power is great indeed. Obe-

*FDA Consumer, April 1973.

sity is regarded as a disease. It affects over 30 million Americans between the ages of 21 to 65, according to the FDA.

Lately, with all the emphasis on exercise and jogging and diets (discussed in Chapter 13), most of us are aware that we are carrying around a lot of excess physical baggage.

Doctor Grant Gwinup, Chairman of the Division of Endrocrinology and Metabolism at the University of California's College of Medicine at Irvine, estimates that we Americans are lugging around something on the order of 5 *billion* pounds of excess blubber.

Author of *Energetics: Your Key to Weight Control,* Dr. Gwinup says, "Our food consumption is going up and our energy expenditure is going down all the time. It is not only unnecessary but quite lethal for a man to accumulate large deposits of fat." (Presumably, the doctor would agree that the danger extends to overweight women also.)

But despite the warnings of distinguished scientists in the field of medicine and nutrition, most of us continue to eat too much and exercise too little, worry about it and, in a moment of minor crisis, finally decide to try one of the "easy-off" preparations either prescribed or dispensed over-the-counter.

As this is being written, the Food and Drug Administration has taken no action against OTC reducing remedies. They are included in the basic categories that are presently under review. But warnings have been sounded to over 600,000 doctors in the United States about preparations available on prescription.

Moreover, the FDA has recommended that the Justice Department, which has the power to regulate certain drugs such as amphetamines and phenmetrazine, broaden its regulations to cover anoretic drugs. This would be done by stringent control of distribution. The Department is already empowered to establish production quotas for any drug that can be abused.

In 1971, recommendations made by the FDA resulted in an 82 percent decrease in the production of amphetamines by pharmaceutical houses producing the drugs for ethical purposes. In 1973, another cut back of 60 percent was recommended. That would mean 60 percent of the 18 percent remaining after the 1971 recommendation. All told, those recommendations add up to a 92 percent reduction in total ethical production of amphetamines since 1972.

As we have seen in earlier chapters, most of the pharmaceutical houses have large manufacturing facilities in foreign countries. It is from these countries that perfectly legitimate production, by foreign standards, become black market importation in the United States of America.

"The problem is enormous, complicated and discouraging," said one FDA official who was reluctant to be identified. In fact, because of the Watergate "fallout," the authors found it difficult to get government employees to speak for the record. Once they were assured that we were not 'spies' with some ulterior political motive, they spoke freely enough and much good information was elicited—"but please don't quote me by name." Since, considering Washington, D.C.'s present political climate, to do otherwise might jeopardize useful careers, we have honored those requests.

The FDA's Neuropharmacological Drug Division has done a very impressive research job evaluating anoretic drugs. The latest techniques, including computer readouts, were employed. All the well-known drugs were reappraised both as generic drugs and as trade name products.

So extensive was the reevaluation that several new drugs soon to be marketed in the United States were also examined. The result is a new set of labeling requirements for anoretic drugs that will warn physicians to use them with extreme caution on a short-term basis only as adjunctive aids in obesity treatments in which the prime factor is diet control.

Anoretic drugs, deemed to have limited usefulness under careful professional supervision, are still available on prescription if the physician, after diagnosing the case, feels they will achieve a good result.

As for the over-the-counter preparations soon to come under the FDA's close scrutiny, they are usually classified in six basic groups despite the fact that their composition and *modus operandi* are considered diverse.

One group claims to achieve appetite suppression by the use of bland bulk-producing agents that fill up the gastrointestinal tract and give one a false sense of fullness.

A second group claims to anesthetize the "hunger center" by the use of benzocaine.

A third group uses glucose, dextrose and other "natural sugars" to satiate the hunger center without the ingestion of large amounts of conventional foods.

A fourth group of OTC weight control preparations uses artificial sweeteners of the sort usually associated with diet drinks.

A fifth group—and perhaps the most popular because of the multimillion dollar educational programs undertaken in the mass media—are canned diet foods that claim to keep one satisfied and well nourished on some 900 calories a day.

And a sixth group employs the chemical phenylpropanolamine to suppress the hunger center. This drug is a pharmacological "first cousin" to ephedrine and amphetamine. In somewhat altered formulation, it is used as a nasal constrictor. But because, in very small doses, it seems to suppress the appetite, it was cleared for use in weight control remedies. In the 1971 AMA's drug evaluation study, the effectiveness of phenylpropanolamine was questioned in the doses usually found in remedies—25 milligrams.

It is required that preparations using the drug warn the user that more than 25 milligrams taken three times daily may be harmful. Certainly the drug should not be used without a physician's approval if the person is suffering from thyroid trouble, heart disease, diabetes, hypertension or any other serious disorder.

Several OTC weight reduction preparations contain combinations of drugs including benzocaine, phenylpropanolamine and caffeine. Abused, they represent a real danger.

No physician interviewed would say that any of the preparations, prescription or proprietary, played any dramatic role in the difficult task of shedding excess fat. It nets down to a question of "pill power" or "will power"; and in the end, will power is the deciding factor.

It is true that some of the preparations taken in combination with diet have a positive psychological effect on the patient. It is often a placebo effect—mind over matter again.

In the short term, our bathroom scale will show some encouraging results. But eventually, it takes a consistent and persistent limiting of balanced food intake to produce permanent results. A few slips and the scales soon confront us with our lapses in the form of added pounds.

Some cases of obesity are due to physiological difficulties. If a serious malfunction of some gland or organ is suspected, the *first* thing he or she should do is see a competent physician. The *last* thing he or she should do is try to handle the problem by self-diagnosis and medication with OTC preparations.

There are a number of cases on record where persons taking benzocaine orally as an appetite suppressant over a protracted period of time became gravely ill. And a number of deaths have been attributed to this sort of self-medication.

At the FDA, one gets the impression that when the OTC weight reduction remedies are finally studied, there may well be some severe restrictions on the use of multiple drugs in a formula.

Jack Spratt could eat no fat;
his wife could eat no lean:
And so betwixt the two of them
they licked the platter clean.

This may be a charming nursery rhyme. And one might reasonably assume that Jack Spratt ended up a widower. In real life, certainly, he would have been following the wiser dietary discipline. Unfortunately because of our very real and unwise life style, it is the men who most often die directly or indirectly of obesity.

One common type of preparation was not included in the most frequently used remedies. That is the *diuretic,* a drug that tends to dehydrate the body by increasing the flow of urine. Called "water pills," diuretic compounds are often advertised as a specific remedy for "pre-period bloat." Persuasive ad copy promises the loss of "pounds and pounds of excess water from all of those puffy places."

Pamabrom and ammonium choloride are two popularly used diuretic compounds. Both are common in menstrual products, although there appears to be no definitive study that substantiates their value for the relief of pre-menstrual tension.

There is evidence, however, that a number of women, reasoning that the loss of pre-menstrual bloat might be extended to general weight loss by the continued use of these OTC preparations, have made themselves ill.

The great danger of protracted use of these preparations—for purposes never intended by the manufacturers—lies in the loss of vital minerals excreted in the urine. No doctor would recommend the use of diuretics for general weight control. One physician said, "If they continue to use those preparations, they'll never have a weight problem—or any other kind of problem. The odds are that in a very short period of time they'll just be plain dead."

So, the inescapable conclusion is simple: while some weight control preparations administered on prescription and under a doctor's observation can be useful in initial weight loss, in the long-run will power and a sensibly planned, sensibly limited food intake is the only safe and sure way to fight the "battle of the bulge"—which brings us to some observations about diets in general.

13 The Great Diet Dupery

From Atkins to Zen, the "fat fighters'" controversy rages; but the ones who are really losing weight are the booksellers, scurrying to keep up with the orders: "Dr. Atkins Diet Revolution"; "The Doctor's Quick Weight Loss Diet"; "Food Without Fads"; "Mirror, Mirror on the Wall"; "The Thin Book by a Formerly Fat Psychiatrist"; "The Expense Account Diet"; "Fat Power"; "Fat Pride"; "The Zen Macrobiotic Diets"; and on and on, apparently ad infinitum!

We counted fifty titles, including the ones usually found only in health food stores. From an admittedly cursory examination of their contents, no two diets seemed alike. But they all shared in common two apparent aspirations: to make their authors a fast buck and to make the readers think that losing blubber can really be as easy as putting it on.

By far, the most controversial of the nutritional and/or diet experts is Dr. Robert C. Atkins whose enormous best seller has motivated several hundred thousand persons to try to take off weight by eating many of the "goodies" other diet experts say are *verboten*.

The Drinking Man's Diet ("Certainly not 'the Thinking Man's Diet'!", observed our physician) achieved great popularity for obvious reasons. The "lose with booze" idea was irresistible to the martini-for-lunch set. As one dieter who tried it said, "I had to give up all those starchy, gooey things I like. But after a few drinks, I didn't give a damn!"

Actually one of the basic tenets of the Drinking Man's Diet was to deprive the dieter of all carbohydrates, presumably except those contained in the alcoholic drinks that were generously permitted. Basically, other than the alcohol, the theory is not too different from Dr. Atkins' whose controversial "fat mobilizing hormone" (FMH/FMS), the existence of which seems to be disputed by a segment of the medical profession, causes excess fat stored in the body to turn into carbohydrates.

It is Dr. Atkins' contention, based on experience with many patients, that as long as one does not ingest carbohydrates, it is possible to eat large amounts of fats and lose weight.

Actually the diet problem has achieved such a "high profile" that the Senate Select Committee on Nutrition and Human Needs, chaired by South Dakota's Democratic Senator George McGovern, opened an inquiry into the whole subject in April 1973. Doctor Atkins turned out to be the star witness. A run down of the partial transcript seems to indicate that Dr. Atkins "gave as good as he got."

The committee was zeroing in on fad diets and it was no coincidence that the Atkins diet was the "head duck in the Senate shooting gallery" on opening day. The committee's objective was to find some practical way to alert the public about the possible dangers in certain fad diets. It will not be easy to accomplish because no legal machinery presently exists that is broad enough in scope to encompass what some legal opinion feels is perilously close to government censorship of reading matter.

James Rowen, a consultant to the Select Committee, admitted that the committee does not know whether the FDA can actually exercise any authority in the area:

> Since most medical products are stringently regulated by the FDA, could a commercially sold diet plan fall under this authority in any way? For example, should we require that a diet plan, since it affects nutritional intake, have a notice affixed to it advising people to see a physician before starting it? There is absolutely no mechanism now for bringing to the public's attention the fact that these could be dangerous.

Concurring in this opinion was Gary Yingling of the FDA who confirmed that the broadest possible interpretation of the administration's regulations would not include such authority. John Walden, also of the FDA, was quoted in the press as saying:

> We're involved in the safety and wholesomeness of products, not censorship. The limit of our authority in the area of weight reduction really applies only to drugs. We've just brought out restrictions on the kinds and amounts of amphetamines marketed, but that's about as far as it goes. Nothing in our laws would stretch to cover the regulation of diet books.

Moreover, Mr. Walden did not seem certain that the FDA authority should be that broad. As expected, Dr. Atkins agreed on the grounds that such censorship would amount to a violation on rights guaranteed in the First Amendment.

The Council on Foods of the American Medical Association seemed to have few, if any, reservations about what should be done to protect the public health, whether the "remedies" be packaged in pills, potions, capsules or between the covers of a book urging what the council regards as unsound medical procedure. .

Doctor Atkins' book was labeled by the council as "unscientific and potentially dangerous to health." In a statement on the subject, the AMA said:

> The council is deeply concerned about any diet that advocates an unlimited intake of saturated fats and cholesterol-rich foods. Individuals responding to such a diet with a rise in blood fats will have an increased risk of coronary artery disease and atherosclerosis, particularly if the diet is maintained over a prolonged period.

Republican Senator Percy of Illinois quoted in part from a statement by Dr. Frederick Stare, head of the Department of Nutrition at Harvard University, in which the internationally famous scientist and syndicated newspaper columnist said, "The Atkins' Diet is nonsense. Any book that recommends unlimited amounts of meat, butter and eggs, as this one does, is, in my opinion, dangerous." Then Dr. Stare is reported to have delivered the *coup de grâce* by saying, "The doctor who makes this suggestion is guilty of malpractice."

Doctor Atkins, apparently unruffled by that peer group "prang," countered with a charge that Dr. Stare was merely expressing a personal opinion while his own point of view evolved from work with ten thousand patients.

In exploration of the subject, however, these writers (both of whom should shed a few pounds gained during long hours of sedentary research and typing) found few medical authorities who supported the high-fat, no-carbohydrate theory. Moreover, family experience—admittedly not definitive but certainly, in this case, alarming—seemed to indicate the possibility for trouble, even for one who followed the diet meticulously. A close member of our family in her mid-fifties went on the diet and followed it faithfully, page for page, for over a month. A routine physical examination revealed that she had shed pounds; but her cholesterol count had risen to 290 from a long-time norm of 215. On a nutritionally conventional diet but with decreased intake, she continued to lose and her cholesterol count returned to her "normal."

One of the most respected publications in the medical profession is *The Medical Letter,* a nonprofit publication on drugs and therapeutics, published by The Medical Letter, Inc., 56 Harrison Street, New Rochelle, N.Y. 10810.

In the May 11, 1973, issue, the Atkins diet was described and evaluated. The conclusions reached in *The Medical Letter* represent the consensus of expert medical opinion, often involving fifty or more experts in related fields. No opinion is sent down to editorial unless it represents a clear consensus. Here is what *The Medical Letter* had to say under the heading, "Evaluation":

J. Yudkin and C. W. Carey (Lancet, 2:939, 1960) showed that obese subjects whose dietary carbohydrate intake is rigidly restricted do not increase their intake of protein and fat proportionately. Thus, they lose weight simply by consuming far fewer calories than usual. The ketosis and inhibition of gastric emptying induced by a low-carbohydrate, high-fat diet may help suppress hunger pangs, which could explain why such a diet helps some individuals to lose weight. If the obese subject on the Atkins diet consumes enough protein and fat to compensate for the calories lost by carbohydrate restriction, there is no reason to believe that he will lose weight....

The Medical Letter states that Atkins describes carbohydrate as a "poison" and sugar as an "antinutrient" and that he subscribes to the belief that reactive hypoglycemia is widespread and generally undiagnosed in the United States.

The *Letter* goes on to point out that Atkins gives no references to studies establishing the long-term effectiveness and safety of his diet.*

In a paragraph headed "Adverse Effects," *The Medical Letter* has this to say:

Most diets that promote ketosis are likely to produce fatigue, dehydration and, in some instances, nausea and vomiting, especially in persons who attempt to remain physically active. Atkins' diet may cause an appreciable hyperuricemia, which can precipitate an attack of gout. The starvation-like state induced by a low-carbohydrate, ketogenic diet stimulates release of free fatty acids into the plasma; in patients with cardiovascular disorders such as cerebrovascular and coronary artery disease, increased free fatty acids may induce cardiac arythmias (M. F. Oliver et al., Lancet, 1:710, 1968). Pregnant women should avoid the Atkins diet because chronic ketosis in the mother could adversely affect the fetus.

In one cogent sentence called, "Conclusion," *The Medical Letter* consensus is summed up as follows: "Although it may be effective in some patients, the Atkins diet is unbalanced, unsound and unsafe."

In our own questioning of physicians, we found none who would give the diet an unqualified endorsement although most of the medical men did agree with the FDA that the low-carbohydrate, high-fat diet *might work with*

*Beyond the "10,000 patients" Dr. Atkins has personally studied.

some patients. They also agreed that it should not be undertaken by persons who buy the book and put themselves on the regimen without first consulting their physician and without paying regular evaluation visits to their physicians during the course of the diet.

In fairness to Dr. Atkins, he would also prefer that the regimen be done under the watchful eye of the physician although he does make provision for the dieter to monitor the ketones in the urine with a simple home "dip stick" test.

It is not likely that the Atkins brouhaha is going to "go away," for the doctor has many disciples and his book continues on the paperback best seller lists as of this writing (February 1974). If it turns out that Dr. Atkins is indeed an avant-garde physician who is "into a whole new thing that works" as some claim, he will not be the first medical man to suffer the lancet wounds of his peers.

Meanwhile, the consensus of conservative medical opinion still obtains with most thoughtful patients: *There are other ways to lose weight that are demonstrably effective and safe.* The trouble is with human nature. We take decades to put on the blubber and then look for some abracadabra to take it off with little or no effort on our part. Patently stupid, we are. But haven't we usually been where our well being involves some personal sacrifices?

From Atkins' diet revolution to Zen macrobiotic diets is a leap clear across the physiological and philosophical spectra. Because most of the intervening ideas are deemed innocuous, foolish and/or generally harmless, *Pray Your Weight Away, Slumberslim* (Sleep Off Your Fat), *The Candy Diet, The Expense Account Diet* (Caviar and Champagne), *The Lovers' Diet* ("Reach for a Mate Instead of a Plate"), *The Grapefruit Diet* and a dozen others, the medical profession has concerned itself mainly with those extremes they regard as physiologically dangerous. High on the list is the Oriental "health diet" known as the "Ohsawa Zen Macrobiotic Diet." It was originated by a Japanese, Georges Ohsawa who died in 1966 in Paris where he lived most of his life.

Such was the popularity of his pseudo-philosophical-physiological persuasion that an Ohsawa Foundation was established in New York City. In the fall of 1968, the FDA confiscated several thousand dollars worth of "health foods" and charged the foundation with perpetrating false and misleading claims to prevent and treat such diseases as anemia, apoplexy, arthritis, cancer and a clutch of other ailments.

The Ohsawa Foundation immediately added to California's reputation as a haven for "off-beat everything" by letting it be known that it was moving to Los Angeles. When the authors attempted to contact the group, no trace could be found under its original name. But there is no problem in finding devotees and disciples by the hundreds among the food-faddist younger set who haunt the health food stores.

Following is an accurate transcript of a casual conversation with one such disciple, a twenty-three-year-old college student complete with long hair, beaded headband, beard, bare feet and a zealot's preoccupation. The encounter took place over a nonbiodegradable plastic cup of organic carrot juice in a health food center patronized by young people in Laguna Beach, California:

ZEN *(pointing to juice):* Man, you're into it, aren't you?

LFC *(puzzled):* I'm sorry, friend—into what?

ZEN: Into the Zen macrobiotic way.

LFC *(a bit apologetically):* I didn't realize I was. I usually have some carrot juice or papaya juice every day. I didn't know I was doing the Zen thing. What is it?

ZEN: Oh man! It's far out. It's the way! Like, it's a religion and diet all in one bag.

LFC: You mean like prayer and fasting as Jesus preached?

ZEN: Wow! Not Jesus, man. Buddha. You know—Zen Buddhism? Like it's an Oriental philosophy for living. A master named Ohsawa learned it from the monks and wrote some books. It's in the books.

LFC: You mean he recommends carrot juice as spiritually uplifting?

ZEN: Not just carrot juice. Any organic food. You know.
...Like when you start, you eat just about anything you
want—as long as it's organic—except meat of course. If
you don't have the spiritual thing, you know, like the "inner strength," you can eat meat for a while—and soups
and vegetables and salads and all fresh stuff like that. Especially fruit.

LFC: What happens when you're ready to give up meat?

ZEN: You just "turn off" on animal food and get into vegetables and fruit and cereals. Especially cereals. When you
go through all the steps you end up just eating cereals.
That's when you've been through Yin and Yang and
reached super consciousness. You only need cereals.

LFC: You mean like Wheaties and Grape-nuts and corn
flakes?

ZEN: Wow! No way! That's artificial. You've got to eat—like—
granola. Only natural stuff. Brown rice is best though,
with the husks left on. That is what the real Zen masters
eat. I mean, like the Buddhists—the ones who can move to
the next plane.

LFC: But don't you need some animal proteins and green
vegetables and yellow vegetables and fruit to make a balanced diet?

ZEN: No, man. When you've advanced to the seventh diet
you don't need anything but the natural cereals. You tran-
scend. You never have to worry about being sick again—
no cancer, no heart attacks, no allergies or anything.
You're purified, man! Your spirit is—like "right on" with
(breaking off and pointing heavenward)—with the—you
know....

LFC *(nodding):* "Like" you've reached a state of grace? Is that it?

ZEN: Wow! Right on. Like you've got it made with God.

The conversation turned to health foods again and LFC
pointed to a 5-pound can of "organic honey" that was "guaranteed free of harmful chemicals—unstrained, unpasteur-
ized, just as nature and the busy bees made it."

LFC: What about this honey?

ZEN: You can use it in Diet Three.

LFC: Is there such a thing as "organic" honey? I mean, how can they keep the bees from straying over to blossoms that have been sprayed with chemicals? How can they be sure?

ZEN *(seriously):* Man, they've got special fields of flowers—like safflower and clover and orange blossoms and they've got them all screened in—like with giant window screens so the bees don't get any pollen but the pure stuff. *(pointing to one of the clerks)* Ask her. She'll tell you.

LFC, this author, who was raised on a ranch and knows about bees, having tended fifty hives, resisted asking the amused clerk, a retired R.N., whom he has known for thirteen years and with whom he exchanges good natured banter about the whole "health food" gambit. Instead he went to the medical library of the University of California at Irvine to see what the non-Buddhist physicians had to say about macrobiotic diets.

What they had to say was not surprising. The AMA's Council on Foods and Nutrition, reviewing the late Georges Ohsawa's philosophy and "medical disciplines" as set forth in his two books, "Zen Macrobiotics" and "The Philosophy of Oriental Medicine" found little to recommend. Following are some excerpts from *JAMA,* October 18, 1971:

> The macrobiotic diet represents an extreme example of a general trend toward natural and organic foods. One of the reasons given for the popularity of these unusual diets is that they are considered to be a means of creating a spiritual awakening or rebirth....

The article suggests that some persons have taken up the Zen diet as an act of defiance, feeling that the "establishment" is personified in the food industry. Others may have turned to the natural or organic diets as an act of protest against war.

It is the consensus of the authors that whatever the motive for embracing the philosophy and its regimen, macrobiotics constitute a major public health problem and are dangerous to its adherents....

Following an objective description of the *modus operandi* of the Zen macrobiotic diet, *JAMA* states:

> Individuals who persist in following the more rigid diets of Zen macrobiotics stand in great danger of incurring serious nutritional deficiencies, particularly as they progress to the highest level of dieting.
>
> Cases of scurvy, anemia, hypoproteinemia, hypocalcemia, emaciation due to starvation and other forms of malnutrition, in addition to loss of kidney function due to restricted fluid intake, have been reported, some of which have resulted in death.

Contrary to the oft expressed, uninformed opinion that the American Medical Association is part of the "prejudiced establishment," the *JAMA* article acknowledges that persons who depart from conventional nutritional practices may unjustly be accused of being food faddists. "There is no doubt that some of these philosophies provide satisfying emotional, spiritual and physical experiences for their followers," says *JAMA* in a display of fair-mindedness not often found in some of the so-called "liberal" publications.

The Council on Foods and Nutrition is unwilling to categorize all unusual dietary philosophies as "hazardous" without first evaluating their nutritional contributions. "But, when a diet has been shown to cause irreversible damage to health and ultimately to lead to death," says the *JAMA* article, "it should be roundly condemned as a threat to human health. The Council on Foods and Nutrition believes that such is the case with the rigid dietary restrictions placed on the followers of the Zen macrobiotic philosophy."

In February 1973, in his syndicated newspaper column, Dr. Walter Alvarez of the Mayo Clinic reported on the case of a young woman who followed the Zen macrobiotic diet faithfully for nine months.

Hospitalized, she died despite heroic efforts to save her. When an autopsy was performed, the pathologist found she had literally died of emaciation due to starvation. Investigation proved that she had eaten nothing but natural cereals, had taken as little water as possible and had eaten sesame seeds and so-called "sea salt."

Doctor Alvarez estimates that the Zen macrobiotic diets, or variations of them, are being followed by at least ten thousand persons, mostly young people on college campuses. The authors' own investigations would not only tend to support that estimate but term it conservative.

One of the most popular of the new natural diets is really an old one. It was advocated back in Egyptian times or quite possibly earlier. It is the vegetarian diet or, as some people now call it, "the legume regimen."

There are degrees of devotion to this dietary fad. Some persons are lacto-vegetarians who include most dairy products in their diets. Some are lacto-ovo-vegetarians who also include eggs in their meals. And then there are the "vegans" or "pure" vegetarians who eschew anything but strictly natural vegetable food and usually prefer it raw or juiced.

Most doctors do not get alarmed if a patient decides to spend a few days on a vegetarian diet, especially if the person compromises and becomes a pro tempore lacto or lacto-ovo-vegetarian, for this ensures at least some of the important nutrients—usually amino acids and vitamin B_{12} that will be largely missing in the strict vegetarian diet.

If the pure vegetarian diet is pursued for a considerable length of time, some severe and potentially dangerous nutritional deficiencies will almost certainly result. A number of health food faddists have argued this point, saying that soy beans, lentils and certain seeds will supply all the basic nutrients needed. But medical persons and qualified nutritionists disagree.

The body cannot synthesize certain critical amino acids. If they are not obtained through a balanced diet, the body soon becomes deficient in them. The names of these vital substances are not too familiar to the average person but they should be if one is trying to plan a well-balanced diet. *Isoleucine, leucine, lysine, phenylalamine, methionine, threonine, tryptophan, valine* and *histidine* are amino acids that must be obtained through intake of certain foods.

Meat, fowl, fish, milk and eggs supply all of them. But any vegetable the faddist may put on his diet list will be lacking in one or more of these essential amino acids. One of the great dangers in the all-cereal Zen macrobiotic diet is the lack of *lysine*. Soybeans and the seed oils are low in *methionine*; so are lentils, peas and beans. They are also deficient in *tryptophan*. And one of the most popular of the "nuts," peanuts, are deficient in both *lysine* and *methionine*.

Nutritionists concede that some vegetable combinations—of unusual variety, generally not obtainable in markets—possibly can supply most if not all the essential amino acids. But there is no question that a diet composed exclusively of commonly used vegetables, unsupplemented by a good variety of fresh fruit, will be deficient in essential amino acids.

Present nutritional research has not yet established just what combinations of vegetables will dependably supply the entire necessary spectrum of amino acids. Therefore it becomes a chancy thing to contrive a do-it-yourself vegetarian diet and put your health in the "laps of the Gods" or at the mercy of some sincere but too seldom scientifically trained "natural food experts" who dispense their dubious wisdom in health food stores and juice bars.

In past works, the authors have been accused of being harsh on such places. There is some justification in the charge when it is made by those health food counsellors who undertake to diagnose and prescribe for customers who come in and ask "What do you have that is good for this and that ailment?" On the other hand, we happily patronize the juice bars and often buy products from the whole grain shelves because we enjoy them and do not mind paying a premium for those we find useful because of sound nutritional values. Too often some of the counsel we have received has come perilously close to quackery, a subject to be discussed in a subsequent chapter.

Unless there is some proved physiological malfunction, the obesity problem nets itself down to our changing life style. Too many of us eat too much and exercise too little. In the lower socioeconomic groups, the situation may well be reversed. A large segment of the population may, in fact, work too much and eat too little—of the proper foods. Among the poor and the old existing on limited incomes, diets are heavy in carbohydrates and other fattening foods—pastas, breads, soft drinks and the like.

Nutritionists fight to change the eating habits at the school levels but admit that with coin-operated food and drink dispensing machines franchised into school cafeterias and in adjacent stores, their task is nearly hopeless.

"Basic nutrition should be a required subject in schools from the first grade on," said one frustrated nutritionist. "We should teach good nutrition like the Catholics teach religion—and with the same fervor. You can't save a soul unless you start with the body it inhabits!"

Doctor Rudolf Noble, co-director of the Hospital Obesity Clinic at the University of California, San Francisco, is certain that the incidence of obesity will increase in direct proportion to the rising cost of meats and other high protein foods. He finds obesity among children on the increase, especially among high school students in the low income groups who consume much larger quantities of carbohydrates and "junk foods" and who are generally more sedentary than they used to be.

A high school athletic coach, who asked not to be named but was anxious to be quoted, said this, "I have one hell of a time fielding a good football team now. The kids are as big as they used to be but now they have more blubber than muscle than they did even five or six years ago. And they run out of steam in practice. God knows they run out of steam during the games. Look at our record so far—aught for seven!"

When asked the reason for the obesity and low energy level, he replied:

Because they aren't eating properly. They eat that ———— that comes out of those vending machines: stale candy bars and peanuts and cokes. That's lunch for a lot of them. The same money spent in the school cafeteria—or even at McDonald's or the Jack-in-the-Box would get them a better meal. Too much starch. Too much sugar. And too much just plain sitting on their fat asses! Even their old men have sense enough to get some protein and jog around the track after work. But not these kids. It's very discouraging.

Not all of the scientific community seems to be as worried about obesity as the physicians we've quoted, or for that matter our harrassed high school athletic coach.

Some nutritionists feel that our preoccupation with obesity is exaggerated and unrealistic and that insurance companies are partially to blame with their average height-weight-age charts.

"There is no such thing as an 'average man or woman,' " they say. "The whole thing started with a reasonable premise but it's gotten out of hand. A billion dollar industry has been built on reducing pills and machines and diets."

One physician charges that the advertising industry, urged on by clients, has refined with diabolical efficiency techniques for selling us "anxiety over our weight."

Part of our bodily structure may be genetically "okay" according to the physician. We may have inherited big bones and heavy muscles. By the "tables" we may be grossly overweight. But a physical examination will show very little excess fat. Heavyweight fighters and football players would probably measure up as dangerously overweight on those charts even though they are in superb physical condition. On the other hand, an insurance executive who happens to fit the chart precisely may, in fact, be dangerously loaded with excess fat.

Doctor Ancel Keys, emeritus professor of the University of Minnesota expressed the opinion before a conference sponsored by the National Institute of Health in October 1973, that "much of the propaganda about overweight goes far beyond scientific justification...."

That brings us to what one physician calls "the ultimate idiocy"—fasting. If cutting down on our intake results in a little weight loss over the short term, why not cut out eating altogether for a while and lose a lot of weight? The reasoning logics well but as we stated earlier, it is possible to be logical without being correct.

What one wants to do in weight control is lose excess fat. But if one resorts to a fasting regimen that extends over a period of weeks—even under doctor's care and in the hospital or under "hospital conditions"—when the body has taken what energy it can from the excess fat and has used it all up, it next begins to draw glucose needed for the central nervous system from the protein in the body, from the muscles and from the liver. In short, you are now no longer losing fat, you are losing the essential you!

That engaging, often overweight television star, Jackie Gleason, may joke about going to the hospital and "fasting" to lose weight. But he didn't go to the hospital just because it was more comfortable there or because he was under surveillance and couldn't cadge a cream puff or a little of his favorite "sauce." He went there to be put on a carefully controlled medical regimen.

Those who can afford to go through that discipline can come out in a week or two looking as "svelt" as the amiable Jackie. But to arbitrarily begin fasting as some labor leaders and protesters have done can be a dangerous self-prescription.

Fortunately, nature has provided some safeguards such as fainting, dizziness and nausea that remind us dramatically that we're going too far. But all in all, most medical men and women advise against a self-imposed fast. "It's far better to slow down on the food," they advise.

Again, the safest course is the cautious one.

14 The Innocent Bystanders: Unborn Children

George Kenneth is only seventy-two hours old. And he's a confirmed "junkie." He was born a junkie. As a matter of medical fact, infant George was a "head" while he was still in his young mother's womb—"hooked" on the drugs she took to quiet the nausea that troubled her from time to time, hooked on the codein in the headache-and-pain-killer compound she had obtained legally in Mexico after a third prescription refill was denied her in San Diego.

Infant George Kenneth is only one of several hundred thousand infants born each year to mothers who are narcotic addicts or who innocently abuse a number of drugs, some available over-the-counter, that act as pain suppressors or tranquilizers.

Each of their infant "innocent bystanders" is doomed to go through the horrors of withdrawal; and if the parents are not aware—and they are usually too preoccupied with satisfying their own habit-hungers—the child may die. At best, it may be physiologically and psychologically "crippled" for life. A few infants are fortunate enough to get into the hands of concerned doctors in clinics where the withdrawal symptoms are recognized and treated. Many infants born to known addicts are usually cared for in foster homes where they get at least "half a shot" at a normal life.

Infants born into "good families," born of mothers who have made their own pregnancies easier with medication, without thinking about or understanding the possible consequences on the unborn child, are usually under the care of perceptive family physicians. Even so, if the mother is taking medication surreptitiously, there is little a suspicious obstetrician can do short of elaborate tests and a medical "third degree" each visit. Questions notwithstanding, there is no guarantee that the pregnant woman will "come clean" and admit that she's been sneaking a few grams of this and that to make things easier. And so, with a handicap, "Baby" Jane Doe or "Baby" John Doe begin what will probably be, at best, a tough, competitive race to achieve in our success-oriented society.

"Baby Mary" appeared normal at birth—the "spitting image of her grandmother who is a very beautiful woman." The young parents are delighted, beam at the compliments of friends, make all of those cooing noises, sing the usual off-key "Rockabye" rhymes and "can hardly wait" until little Mary begins to talk.

But Baby Mary will never talk. She has no way to learn. She was born deaf because her mother had taken courses of streptomycin for several "infections" during pregnancy.

Other babies such as little Mary whose mothers had taken quinine near the time of birth also share the risk of being born with impared hearing. Apart from the trauma experienced by the parents—the guilt and self-castigation (and anxiety about adding to the family)—there will be the financial burden of special schooling and the too often hopeless quest for surgical correction of the malfunction or deformity.

Baby X is a "thing"—hardly a human—a cretin, a tragic little spirit doomed to imprisonment in a defective body because its mother, during her pregnancy, had taken progesterone to stop a condition diagnosed as functional uterine bleeding.

So frightened was she by the appearance of blood "when none should appear" that she arranged to get prescriptions refilled through a friend who was also taking the drug that affects the functioning of endocrine glands. Later, under questioning, it was learned that she had taken the drug intermittently for six of the nine months of her pregnancy.

Less dramatic, perhaps, but still distressing is the warning to pregnant women that the administration of hormones—

progestins and testosterone—during gestation can virilize the external genitalia of the female fetus.*

Preparations containing iodides have been shown to damage or destory the thyroid gland in the developing fetus when the medicine is taken during the first third of the pregnancy term. Congenital goiter and hypothyroidism have also been attributed to preparations containing iodides.

One might say, "Well, those are strong prescription drugs. Things could happen if you abuse them." And that is true. But it is also true that all sorts of neonatal (newly born) difficulties are possible with such simple OTC items as ascorbic acid, vitamin C.

As unlikely as it may seem, there are literally hundreds of cases on record where scurvy developed in infants whose mothers had been taking unusually large doses of ascorbic acid and other vitamins in an effort to make certain the developing child would have a "good start" prior to birth.

What happened, the doctors deduced, was unexpected but understandable: the child, once born, was removed from the source of vitamins in its mother's bloodstream. Because the vitamin was not supplied after birth, the infant actually developed a deficiency that resulted in scurvy. A pregnant woman following the advocates of extremely high doses of vitamin C as protection against the common cold—especially a woman who is prone to catching colds—might very well find her newborn child developing symptoms of vitamin C deficiency once it has been deprived of its prenatal source.

It is possible that the child will receive some of the vitamin from the mother if she continues to take it and the child is breast fed—a practice that is no longer as common as it was several generations ago.

Antihistamines have long been suspected as a possible danger drug if administered during the first three months of pregnancy. While there seems to be little evidence that *meclizine* and *cyclizine* and several other antihistamines

*The Medical Letter, vol. 19, no. 6, Issue 344, March 17, 1972.

are to blame for abnormalities, tests have shown that they do produce severe deformities in laboratory animals. Most doctors would not prescribe antihistamines to pregnant women since over the long term tests the produce positive (bad) results in lab animals often are capable of creating the same problems in humans.

Barbiturates are another source of possible neonatal problems. If taken by a pregnant woman who is nearing the end of her term, or if administered during labor to depress her central nervous system and make the ordeal of birth easier, the medication can produce serious respiratory problems in the newly born child.

Ideally, no medication should be administered to a pregnant woman except under the strictest supervision of the physician. Moreover, if she has been dosing herself with various OTC preparations and the physician does not query her, she should volunteer the information and give the doctor the brand name of the product in order to conduct a careful check on the active ingredients in that particular formula.

Earlier, we discussed the possibility of dangerous interaction between the ingredients in various drugs. A physician who has kept abreast of new developments will know about these drugs. If the obstetrician does not, a consultation with a pharmacist is in order. Also, in the unlikely event that the physician is not up to date, he or she may very quickly check a number of publications, among them the *Handbook of Non-Prescription Drugs* for the current year.

Doctors particularly warn against the use of preparations containing amphetamines during pregnancy. Here again, tests have proved that the drug can produce serious abnormalities in laboratory animals and therefore have the potential to create problems in human fetuses. These anoretic drugs, (appetite suppressors) have a very short term effectiveness and have been shown to create what amounts to withdrawal symptoms in children and adults who have used them for weight control.

Recently, fenfluramine, an amphetamine derivitive, has been substituted as an appetite suppressor. Many doctors feel that since it is a closely related chemical substance it too should be ruled out for use by pregnant women.

The one thing many obstetricians say pregnant women should remember, and bear in mind continually during their pregnancy, is that the mother and the fetal child are inseparable, one and the same thing; but it does not necessarily follow that medication that helps the mother will not harm the unborn child. On the contrary, as research shows, anything strong enough to relieve an adult symptom has the potential of doing tragic damage to the fetus.

We have only to remember the thalidomide tragedies, a drug regarded as thoroughly tested and safe for use in Germany and other European countries, to see what can result when a pregnant woman "takes the latest discovery" to allay her nausea or her headaches or any of the other discomforts that beset a woman who is "carrying."

The little "innocent bystanders" have no protection from external threats to new life except that which is intermittently provided by the physician, and the continuing common sense precautions taken by the mother-to-be. For a pregnant woman, even a little medication may prove to be too much for her unborn child. The medicine may not result in actual physical deformity or impairment of the child; but it may well result in some undetected weakness or malfunction that, in later years, can become a very real detriment. Nobody will argue for long that the first blessing the parents can give their offspring is the strongest possible physical equipment that expertly applied science and genetic inheritance can provide.

15 Duck the Quacks!

The year was 1933. The place was the old Hollywood Women's Club at the corner of Hollywood Boulevard and La Brea Street. The occasion was the weekly broadcast of the *Hollywood Barn Dance,* starring the Crockett Family, The Stafford Sisters (Jo was the little kid in the middle), Sheriff Loyal Underwood and the Arizona Wranglers with special guitar solos by Joe Bishop and comedy by rolly-polly former circus acrobat and silent pictures stooge for Lloyd "Ham" Hamilton, Buddy Duncan ("This belly cost me a hundred thousand in restaurants!").

The show was one of the most popular on station KNX, now the Columbia Broadcasting System's key station in the West, but then owned by the Western Broadcasting Company with studios on the Paramount Pictures "lot."

As it was with many of those early "country and western" radio shows, sponsors participated (bought spots) in quarter hour segments. The station's primary nighttime coverage area was the eleven western states; but KNX, because of its clear channel, had a phenomenal DX factor—which means that its nighttime signal reached halfway around the world—quite literally.

The sponsors remembered most clearly were Peruna, Kester Metal Mender, Cogoin, Krazy Water Krystals, Currier's Tablets, Formula Five-Fifteen and Tablet 66.

Of those proprietary remedies, certainly the best known was Peruna, the invention—more properly, the "concoction"—of one Dr. S. B. Hartman, often called just plain

"S. B." by those who discovered that its principal active ingredient was "effective" enough to get it barred from sale on Indian reservations.

Peruna was so famous, so nationally popular, at one dollar a bottle, that its competitors started a ground swell of rumors about it, saying among other things that "the acids and minerals in it will turn your teeth black."

Accordingly, the young announcer, dressed in bib overalls and a straw hat, would walk out on stage and, in his best assumed country accent and with neighborly confidence, would say *(holding up the bottle for the sizable live audience)*:

> Folks, you all know what a wonderful product "Peruny" is, and you know how jealous some of them other so-called medicines git when they see our success. So I don't have to tell you what lies are. You know 'em when you hear 'em. And a lot of lies are bein' told about "Peruny." *(shakes head sadly)*
>
> So what I want to do now is to tell you some plain truth. The competition is just plain old liars when they spread the rumor that you gotta drink Peruny with a straw because it'll turn yore teeth black! *(indignantly)* It jest ain't so! *(showing teeth)* Jes' look at my teeth—and I bin takin' Peruny fer that run-down feelin' fer some time now. And I'm here to tell you that I feel *better!*

The bucolic balderdash went on for two to three minutes and the claims were just outrageous. And the house was packed with "true believers."

The country was still "dry" in those days and there is no question that the announcer did feel better because Peruna's most active ingredient originally was 27 percent pure grain alcohol.

Since the male half of this collaboration was often that "country boy" announcer, he speaks from personal experience. "Peruny" didn't make your teeth black, but the prescribed dose, three wine glasses daily, "shore could make a body feel better."

The Peruna Formula was changed from time to time. At one point in the early 1900s, the Internal Revenue authorities said to Dr. Hartman, "put some real medicine into your drink or open a bar." Doctor Hartman complied promptly by adding two laxitives, senna and buckthorn. The ingredient list on the label, barely legible, made note of the formula change. It seems though that thousands of "run-down" folks, in their haste to feel better, did not bother to read the changes.

Inevitably, there were some ghastly results. Temperance women who had taken their usual daily dose of the new formula suddenly departed the meeting room wearing stricken looks. Business men bolted from meetings, and didn't return to their offices for several days. Doctors who were consulted thought the good people had picked up a strange "germ" and advised taking more Peruna.

This author clearly remembers the disastrous effects being described by his Uncle Wirt who, when he finally found out what was making him "feel better," said, "Hell, if that's all it is, I'll make up a batch myself—without the physic." He did. And he and some of his cronies continued to "feel better" until the Eighteenth Amendment was finally repealed.

As a result, Peruna fell on evil times. The formula underwent several more changes. In the 1930s, it was a fairly innocuous preparation enjoying a national revival due to radio. Its alcoholic content had been reduced slightly to around 17 percent, but it found ready acceptance by the temperance-minded who nonetheless wanted to feel "braced."

Just when the preparation finally disappeared, we do not recall. But we remember some of the lore surrounding the quacks and charlatans of the "patent medicine era." A fictional, though none-the-less instructive story on the topic is H. G. Wells' famous novel *Tono-Bungay*.

The late Stewart Holbrook, in his book "The Golden Age of Quackery" (MacMillan, 1959) recounts in marvelous detail the "infighting" between the patent medicine tycoons, their troubles with the government and with crusading editors and reporters. He recalls among other incidents, the righteous fury of the famed editor of *The Ladies' Home Journal*, Edward Bok, who ran an account of an exposé test of several of the most popular alcoholic remedies.

When equal amounts of the remedies were placed in flasks, heated and the vapors piped to gas lamp mantles, a dose of Peruna kept the lamp 'lit' for two minutes and forty seconds—second only to Hostetter's Celebrated Stomach Bitters which managed to keep the mantle glowing for an even four minutes. It takes little imagination to conjure up a vision of the number of "ailing" men and women who got "lit" and "glowed" for much longer than four minutes while undergoing their own consumer tests. Incidentally, according to Bok, Lydia E. Pinkham's Vegetable Compound kept the test lamp glowing only five seconds less than Peruna. All of which simply proves that these three remedies, as then formulated, richly deserved their popularity as "bracers." The moral back then, as it is today, must have been: "Sin by any other name is just as *sweet* and far easier on the conscience." And if there can be any question about the financial rewards to the purveyors of these nostrums, it is said that Dr. Hartman's partner, Frederick W. Schumacher, left $50 million to the Gallery of Fine Arts in Columbus, Ohio.

The beginning of the end of "the Golden Age" came with the establishment of the Federal Trade Commission in September 1914. The end itself was virtually assured with the establishment of the Federal Communications Commission in 1934. The FTC, alerted to its responsibilities in the matter of advertising, began checking copy claims. The FTC, exercising its power over the uses of radio and later television, began its own policing duties with the result that while honesty in advertising had become the best policy in general, it did not prove to be for the quacks and charlatans. It put most of the old-timers out of business.

The line between "innovative procedures" and "remedies" is a blurred one. Some of the medical miracles in common use today were characterized as "dangerous quackery" only a generation or so ago. Among them was the whole system of immunization by vaccinations. Few are alive today who remember the early furor over smallpox vaccinations. But many adults will remember the commotion that was caused a decade ago by the Salk and Sabin systems of polio immunization when both were called for as "mandatory" in schools. And we have already discussed the fluoridization controversy.

The days of the extravagant claim such as the one made by Peruna that "common catarrh is the cause of all illnesses" are gone. But all such things are relative and so now we find the Food and Drug Administration cracking down almost weekly on remedies and devices that may not actually "spell out" their unwarranted claims but manage to convey them by implication.

It is precisely this abuse, or potential for abuse, that has brought about the basic reevaluation of all OTC drugs and those cosmetics that pretend to be drugs. As troublesome as it may be for manufacturers who are more concerned about earnings per share than they are about sharing their earnings, the American public will soon be one of the best protected bodies in the world. Even so, according to the Council of State Governments in Lexington, Kentucky, the American public is bilked of over $70 *billion* each year.

Just how much of this involves medical quackery is not stated. Quite likely it is not accurately known. The council's figures include such items as home repair, fraudulent furniture sales known as the "bait and switch scam," fraudulent real estate deals,* used car sales abuses and a score of others. But there is little doubt, according to the medical profession, that many of the reducing and "easy does it" exercise devices, particularly the electrical or "magnetic" ones, are of dubious value. Some of the worst of them are now being sold to Americans by companies in Europe and Asia who are doing a mail order business that is difficult to control.

For example, at last count, there were twenty-two phallic-shaped battery vibrators on the market, many made in Hong Kong and Taiwan, that are of highly dubious value—except for some questionable uses alluded to by the "cute" copy writers or by the sensuous appearing nude female models cuddling them with eyes heavy lidded, their moist lips agape with unmistakable orgiastic ecstasy.

*Cooley, *Land Investment, U.S.A.*, Nash, 1974.

There have been many efforts to define quackery. Most have been unsuccessful. The best one found in the authors' research is a definition given by Dr. Samuel R. Sherman at the California Congress on Medical Quackery in San Francisco over a decade ago:

> The problem of quackery, or as it is more carefully designated, 'unproved treatment methods,' is an old and serious one. Approximately one twentieth of all monies spent for medical care is wasted on worthless or harmful forms of treatment. This wastage totals one billion dollars yearly.*
>
> Despite this menacing misuse of money, there has been discouragingly slow progress made in the past fifty years to control the problem. Deplorable as the wastage of money is, more dangerous are the losses of life and health from improper treatment, the creation of false hope, and the prevention of rehabilitation at the proper time....

Doctor Sherman pointed out that one of the difficulties in defining quackery lies in the fact that it is "bordered on one side by incompetent care, and on the other side by legitimate research of the new and unusual."

He felt that care should be taken not to stifle research or prevent that which could hold some promise, and that "motivation" should be considered as a critical factor in the definition. As a demonstration of his own fair-mindedness, Dr. Sherman suggested the following "simple working definition."

> Quackery is the use of discredited or disproved methods, techniques, or theories in the diagnosis and/or treatment of a disease, and where this treatment is given in bad faith or is consistently and considerably below the standards for medical care in the community.

Displaying a fine sense of history, Dr. Sherman observed that the California Medical Association has been concerned

*Some estimates say two and a half times that now.

with quackery for many decades. He pointed out that one of the motives for organizing the early medical societies in California was to control the untrained, unprincipled and self-appointed quacks who were attracted to California during the Gold Rush in 1849-1850.

"These early-day charlatans linger on in a few television westerns," he observed, "but in real life they have been replaced by more sophisticated and subtle persons."

Several medical persons have attempted to list the "symptoms" of quackery. Doctor Walter Alvarez made a list of "Thirteen Hints on How To Spot a Quack."

Doctor Sherman boiled it down to seven danger signs: Beware, he implied, if the drug or the device:

1. is generally secret,

2. is advertised,

3. is limited to one proponent (or is so implied),

4. is poorly documented (clinical and other records are incomplete or absent),

5. is most highly praised by those who are least qualified in this particular area of judgment (politicians and *authors* (!) are often cleverly used by quacks),

6. or its proponent is "persecuted by the medical trust," usually the AMA,

7. is often a discarded orthodox drug or form of therapy. It has been stated that quacks are generally fifty years behind in their theories and correctness of thought—but not in their advertising and psychology. (The control of quacks is more archaic than are the ideas of quacks and their supporters.)

But the doctor adds that despite the universality of these characteristics, quacks differ greatly; and each must be carefully studied for effective control.

Perhaps no group of persons in this world is more susceptible to quackery and the blandishments of charlatans than those suffering from cancer and rheumatoid arthritis. As soon as the nature of the disease is medically confirmed, they realize they quite probably have been sentenced to ćeath or to a life of painful suffering.

Honest physicians feel they must tell their patients what the prognosis is and the truth can be terrifying. Since the medical profession attempts to be unvaryingly honest about these diseases and its ability to cure them or to arrest them, the door is left wide open, in many cases, for the charlatan to come in with his confident promises.

The list of miracle "cures" is long indeed. It includes everything from special Argentine serums taken from a sick horse to the essence of a fruit pit. Moreover, a number of distinguished women and men—some of them medical doctors (and, we confess, a few "distinguished authors *and* editors") have been and still are among the strongest advocates of several controversial cancer and arthritis cures. Their support is based on what they honestly feel are good results demonstrated on themselves, family members or good friends. They tend to pay little attention to the sound clinical conclusion that cancer is not just "one disease" but is actually an infinitely complicated physiological phenomenon. Many forms of cancer appear to have little in common beyond the uncontrolled proliferation of "wild cells."

It is a well-established fact that in certain people, for reasons not entirely understood even by the most advanced cancer researchers, there will be a sudden remission for no apparent cause. It can be, and often is, attributed to one of the "miracle cures" that the desperate patient has resorted to when conventional medical procedures were found to be unsatisfactory.

Often we hear the complaint that such patients are "driven" into the arms of the charlatans because of the ultraconservatism of the medical establishment. "They test promising new things to death while patients continue to die!" is one of the most frequently heard charges.

"The only sensible response to that," commented an FDA official, "is to remind them of the thalidomide tragedy that resulted because a new medicine was not 'tested to death.' "

But memories are short and charges are still being heard on radio and television and in the press that the Food and Drug

Administration has built up a great self-serving bureaucracy—that its claims of being understaffed are not valid because they stem from a top-heavy T.O. (table of organization) that is the result of unrealistic precautions and procedures.

Critics of the FDA cite the record time in which England and France and Germany get new drugs approved for human use. These same critics ignore the thalidomide horror that, but for the FDA's system of checks and balances, could have resulted in thousands of grotesquely deformed children here. (More on the FDA's role in protecting us in the following chapter.)

Quack-ism is still rampant in this country. The worst of it seems to be confined to the reducing and cosmetic and health food fields. Thanks to protective laws, much of it is relatively harmless to the person of the victim, if not to his purse.

Each of us has deep needs and aspirations. Each of us has a self-image and most of us have an ideal that we somehow fall short of. Some of us would like to be older, younger, fatter, slimmer, more hirsute, more muscular, sexier—and so it goes.

These "mitty-ish" daydreams are cleverly exploited by men and women who are skilled practical psychologists. They understand the subjective as well as the objective appeal of any product or system that promises to achieve our fondest aspirations for ourselves—no matter how weasel-worded their advertising appeals must be.

So we spend hundreds of millions on gadgets, gimmicks and gunk, all of which manage to skirt, avoid or minimally comply with the advertising and labeling regulations designed to protect us—not from the charlatans—*but from ourselves.* And that is the crux of the problem.

We read of some new remedy or appliance in the press. Even though the qualifying paragraphs are present in the piece, the real story lies in the *promise* of some miracle medicine or medical mechanism.

Those who are suffering from a malady or malaise or imaginary personal deficiency read and their hopes soar. If the imminent miracle happens to be a medicine for one of the major ailments, a great hue and cry can rise that may actually bring abou' premature approval, if sufficient political pressure is applied.

According to one distinguished physician who asked to remain unnamed:

> Perhaps there is less charlatanism in clinical medical practice today than there is in one branch of our profession—psychiatry. We are flooded with books these days on dozens of behavioral theories. There is no regulation on these because there are no practical professional parameters. Anybody with a plausible theory on human behavior that can be supported with so-called authoritative quotes and a few questionable case histories can find a clientele. In my opinion—and we get some of the physical manifestations of these psychological wrecks—this is a particularly pernicious form of quackery. Often these theories are tried out on desperate patients who are literally on the ragged edge, mentally. We have seen therapy make wrecks of people. Several cases have become addicts, totally dependent on psychoactive drugs that "padded" them and kept them facing reality.

The physician, speaking one evening in his home, went on to say that it was not his purpose to indict any branch of his profession:

> In all fairness I must say that many of the physical wrecks were the result of therapy by improperly or inadequately trained psychotherapists some of whom were self-appointed and held no valid degrees.
>
> If you and Mrs. Cooley had a plausible theory about human behavior, there is no law I know of that would prevent you from holding informal group therapy sessions or encounter groups. I do not mean this personally because you two are mature people—writers with a deep understanding of human nature—but it would be possible for you, or someone less qualified, even with a degree, to initiate a totally distorted behavior pattern in people that, in time, could result in all sorts of antisocial behavior. Some such behavior could have the potential for violence and real danger. But there would be nothing to prevent you from hanging out your "shingle" and writing a "best seller."

By the same token, if you had a pet nutrition theory—a sort of potpourri of Adele Davis, Gaylord Hauser, Carleton Fredericks and a half dozen others, you could publish your notions, claim that you had tested them on scores of people over the years and attract a following.

You can double-talk and imply and hint and half promise that your particular system of nutrition has been beneficial in relieving the misery of this and that ailment and nobody can lay a glove on you.

Last week we operated on a man in his mid-fifties whose colon was literally riddled from eating a special "natural cereal" concoction put together by a friend. The man had diverticulosis and the high bran and fibre content of the unrefined grains, coconut, sunflower and sesame seeds had literally scratched through his gut and sent him into peritonitis.

There is no way the public can be protected against such folly except through intensive educational programs. As I've said many times, I'd like to see nutrition taught as a required subject from the first grade on. So would you if you saw the medical disasters we see in the operating rooms every day.

The home-made formula sounded very much like those in the new "old-fashioned" health cereals so popular these days. We asked this physician if such food was generally dangerous:

Not necessarily. They are usually safe for healthy young, active people; but I would not recommend them for older sedentary people. Generally, some roughage is desirable for almost everybody. But it doesn't have to be harsh roughage such as bran. That is a virtually indigestible substance. In any case, roughage should be thoroughly chewed. All food should be, just to make certain that the first phase of the digestive process has been properly initiated. But one should be especially careful to chew brans, nuts, coconut and all substances containing small seeds, particularly raisins. And let us not forget popcorn. In a normal gut, well-chewed roughage can be beneficial and a help to peristalsis. But you'd better make damned good and sure you've got good teeth and perfect plumbing before you start on one of those diets. You can die unnaturally from the wrong kinds of natural food!

The only way, then, that one can "duck the quacks" is to apply that primary precaution of precautions, common sense. No matter how urgent the need for relief or a cure, in the long run it will be safer—and surer—to play the odds. And the odds are that conservative medical opinion will be right more often than it will be wrong. Certainly it is right when it cautions against the use of untried drugs, medicines or medical procedures. Not always perhaps, but most often, such untried remedies will be advocated by quacks and charlatans or, at the very least, improperly qualified, well intentioned humanitarians.

16 You and the FDA

In the "golden age" of patent medicines and nostrums which extended roughly from the mid 1800s until 1906 when the first Food and Drug Act was passed by congress, it was possible to put almost any ingredient into a "remedy," give it a "high-sounding" or pseudoscientific name and peddle it as a specific remedy for almost all the ailments the human body is heir to—and a number that have never existed and never will.

Opium, morphine, cocaine and alcohol were the standby basic ingredients. To them were added a number of herbal flavorings, sugar preparations and water. Thousands upon thousands of column inches in newspapers and magazines, acres of gaudy signs painted on barns and thousands of "medicine show" pitchmen regaled the public with unabashed claims.

The consequences of this high pressure salesmanship (and a goodly amount of ethical prescription) was a population in which there were tens of thousands of *innocent* addicts. There were no OTC drugs designated as such in those days. Almost everything was over-the-counter. Doctors might well prescribe an opiate for a pain killer—opium and morphine were the workhorse drugs—but the patient, having once been given them could continue to get them in one form or another for as long as it seemed necessary.

Most of the nonaddictive analgesics we take for granted today were not available then. Doctors and quacks, often one and the same, were forced to rely on opiates in one form or another to make patients comfortable.

Heroin, an opium derivative, was discovered in 1874. By 1898 it was manufactured in quantity and was being touted vigorously as *a cure for drug addiction.* By 1920 this country had one addict for each 400 of the population—or approximately 300 for each 100,000 population. This figure compares with approximately 40 addicts per 100,000 of population in 1971 according to the Bureau of Narcotics and Dangerous Durgs. This figure becomes more credible when we realize that today, in this age of instant communication, we are so much more aware of drug use and hear and read about so many "busts." Inevitably, we get the impression that drug addiction is virtually pandemic. (Some sources say this is true of alcohol addiction. Actually, *any* addiction is "too much.")

Much of the drug news involves young people experimenting with "pot," "uppers" and "downers" and LSD. From the figures, it is evident that only a small portion of them actually get "hooked on the hard stuff" and for that we can thank the dedicated staff of the Federal Bureau of Narcotics who fight endlessly against the most appalling odds. Thanks must go also to the Food and Drug Administration, that much maligned and generally misunderstood division of the Department of Health, Education and Welfare, that has grown from a tiny, harrassed group of "agents" in 1906 to a multifaceted organization of scientists and administrators who, despite being a "politically sensitive" group, work daily miracles in guarding the public well-being.

Because the FDA is so generally misunderstood, it is worth tracing the growth of the administration from those early beginnings.

The precursor of the present day Food, Drug and Cosmetic Act was the pioneer Food and Drug Act of 1906.

Though the act marked a great step in the direction of control of harmful products and of standards of quality, particularly in interstate commerce, that early law did not require the manufacturer to make verifiable therapeutic claims on his product labels.

The first attempt at regulating label claims was made in 1912 when Congress passed the Shirley amendment which provided penalties for misbranding.

Because the government had not yet established an agency equal to the task, and since the burden of proving deliberate fraud devolved upon the government, enforcement was limited to the prosecution of those manufacturers who made patently outrageous claims. They were many!

It took one hundred deaths from a sulfanilamide elixir containing diethylene glycol to expand the amended 1906 Act. Even so, under the broadened Food, Drug and Cosmetic Act, passed by Congress in 1938, a manufacturer was only required to prove that a drug *not generally recognized as safe* was shown to be safe *prior to marketing.*

There was still plenty of room for error in this procedure. But it was another step, however small, along the road to the realistic protection of a largely defenseless public through complete labeling. The chief fault lay in the liberal requirements approved by Congress, requirements that were much less stringent than those proposed by the men who had to contend with the problem of protecting the public against harmful drugs.

Essentially the 1938 Act required that the manufacturer fill out a new drug application and submit it for approval. The burden was then on the applicant. The firm produced data purporting to show that the drug was safe for use under the conditions described in the proposed labeling. However, if a drug was generally recognized as safe, no pre-clearance was required.

Political pressure on lawmakers being the effective tool it still is, a "grandfather clause" was written into the 1938 law. Described by a disgusted scientist as "sheer murder," it allowed drugs that had *not been recognized as safe, but which were on the market prior to the enactment of the 1938 law, to continue to be sold to the public providing the article was subject to the 1906 Food and Drug Law.* Moreover, the labeling could be left *unchanged!*

In effect what this "lobbyists' shenanigan" did was exempt from regulation hundreds of potentially dangerous drugs that had met the unrealistic and largely inadequate requirements of that pioneer 1906 law.

Things went along in a manner largely agreeable to the drug industry until the thalidomide tragedy in the late 1950s and early 1960s. Then, in 1962, the late Senator Kefauver conducted a series of hearings on the drug industry in general and on its pricing policies.

The material produced in those hearings resulted in the Kefauver-Harris Bill amending the 1938 Federal Food, Drug and Cosmetic Act. Under the revised laws all new drugs, whether prescription or OTCs, were required to be *proved effective as well as safe prior to marketing.*

But even this new amendment contained a welcome "cop-out" for the pharmaceutical houses who kept continual but subtle pressure on representatives and senators.

The "cop-out" was the word *new*. The amendment required an effectiveness review of all *new* drug products that had been approved for safety between 1938 and 1962, thus permitting the "grandfather clause" to provide an umbrella again for hundreds of *older* products that were *not* recognized as safe, but which had been on the market *prior* to the enactment of the 1938 law, to be peddled unmolested. These machinations shed some light on the meaning of the term "politically sensitive."

The FDA, far from content but grateful for any small gain in the battle to force the makers of drugs and drug products into a position of total responsibility for the safety and quality of their products, enlisted the aid of the National Academy of Sciences, National Research Council, to review some four thousand drugs that fell within the "new drug" category.

The review was conducted by thirty panels of physicians who were recognized as qualified experts in their respective fields. Of the 4,000 products reviewed, 400 were OTC drugs but they represented nearly the entire spectrum of such remedies. *Seventy-five percent of them were found to be ineffective for one or more of their intended uses.**

The FDA, looking at the results which did not particularly surprise its scientists, regarded them as more than sufficient evidence that the entire OTC market should be reviewed. But how to accomplish this practically when the most conservative estimates of the OTC market contains a quarter of a million branded products? (Some "informed" sources put the figure at 500,000!) Moreover, most of these products have never been submitted to the FDA for so much as a label review.

Even though it is estimated that there may be as few as two hundred active ingredients in the entire OTC market, many call for different doses and many are used in combinations that are believed to be potentially dangerous.

If one uses the median figure of 250,000 drugs on the market, and only 25 percent of them are regarded as effective by the NAS-NRC standards, the FDA would have to litigate 187,500 actions. Patently, such an action would require years, even if there were no appeals. Moreover, to embark on such an unrealistic course would require an enormous expansion of certain divisions of the FDA; and the length of time involved to reach judgment would be unfair to the public who might be deprived of an effective OTC during the trial period. It would also be unfair to the manufacturer of such a product.

Earlier, we mentioned that the FDA finally agreed that OTC drugs must be placed in categories and that the only practical way would be to review the drugs in each category collectively. That process is presently underway now. While it may not be regarded as ideal, the system will provide a practical "blanket" review that will evaluate all drugs, except .. and here comes that "grandfather clause" again.

This time, however, the FDA has some clout. Under the law, these products may be regarded as *misbranded*. If that

**Federation Proceedings,* vol. 32, no. 4, April 1973.

is suspected under the new criteria, the FDA may use a new legal approach. If their case stands up, a federal court may find the firm in violation of the 1962 Act and force it to conform by relabeling or changing the formulation.

To counter the temptations inherent in the practice of allowing the drug companies to contract with "independent" testing laboratories whom they pay for producing evaluations of their products, the FDA is submitting the manufacturers' data to their own independent testing organizations. Since the FDA has no commercial stake in the outcome of the evaluations, it is without the prejudice that could normally be expected to be present in the officers of corporations who hire their own experts. "We are not interested in profits," said one FDA official, "just protection."

So, this last step taken by the FDA is a giant one compared to the inching along that has been necessary since 1906, but particularly since 1938. The political pressure is still being applied and the possibility for commercial hanky-panky still exists, mortals being what mere mortals are. But most of the "cop-outs" have been negated now. The FDA frankly says, "this history-making review will have lasting effects on the drug market by eliminating ineffective OTC products and by providing the *consumer with a sound choice of drugs for appropriate self-medication.*"

An example of how this new procedure will work may be gained from a hypothetical example. The case involves a famous brand name protein-vitamin bar which is sold mainly in health food stores and health food sections of supermarkets and drug stores.

Because of its ingredients and the labeling, it is now theoretically regarded as a medicine under the new FDA regulations. Nothing much is going to happen to the many products that presently fall in this theoretical category for several years (we were told anywhere from three to five years) admits the FDA.

But when the evaluation is made the product will have three options:

1. Cut down its "medical" ingredients to 50 percent of the Recommended Daily Allowances fixed by the FDA and sell itself as an ordinary "food" but subject to nutritional labeling.

2. Reformulate its principal "medical" ingredients up to as much as 150 percent of the RDA and present itself as a dietary supplement.

3. Or market itself as an OTC drug product until the review panel on vitamins, minerals and hematinics gets around to classifying that type of product as effective for the prevention or treatment of specific diseases or disorders.

The FDA feels that the consumer will begin to realize some benefits from the new "federal scriptures" sooner than the five years it estimates it will take to finish the reevaluations. The officials feel this will come about because the manufacturers, apprised of the new criteria, will start complying voluntarily. If that proves correct, some of the pharmaceutical houses who have had products and profits pretty much their own way for decades may have cause to reflect on an observation made by Francis Bacon: "Prosperity is the blessing of the Old Testament; adversity is the blessing of the New!"

17 Meditate Before You Medicate

What this book has really been about is human nature and common sense; and the two are often at odds. It is eminently human to want to do everything possible to save ourselves when we find we're in grave danger. This is never more true than when we fear we are seriously ill and the possibility for a cure seems beyond the reach of present medical science.

However, there are other crises, not imminently serious but nonetheless discomforting and disconcerting. It is for relief of these lesser troubles that we most often turn to the OTC drugs. And it is precisely because of our growing, and to a large degree necessary, dependency on these over-the-counter remedies that the federal government, through the Department of Health, Education and Welfare's Food and Drug Administration, has been moved by evidence of widespread abuses (by both customer and manufacturer) to strengthen its regulations.

The FDA does not want to become a surrogate parent, leading us by the hand through the perils of prescription and nonprescription drugs. It has neither the legal right nor the moral obligation to do more than educate both supplier and user to their respective responsibilities.

These are more easily spelled out for the manufacturer— the primary source of ethical and proprietary remedies. That is precisely what has happened with the evaluation of ethical drugs recently completed; and it is the objective of the evaluation of OTC drugs now being conducted by the independent panels of experts.

The FDA officials are under no delusions. They know that no matter how great the strides in checking the safety, effectiveness, purity, uniformity and honesty of labeling the products that will ultimately be evaluated in their respective categories, the final safeguard against abuse must lie with the user of the drug and with those charged with prescribing its use, in the case of "ethical" drugs.

To be practical, these safeguards must be based on the public's knowledge, not so much of the physiological *modus operandi* of the drugs themselves, but of the potential danger that lies in abusing even the most innocuous remedies. This is an on-going educational process and a most difficult one. The doctors themselves must participate in this educational program.

Some time ago when our long-time family physician retired from active practice, the authors found themselves in need of a new "family physician." Since we had moved our residence and had been commuting fifty-five miles to see our old friend and physician, we sought to find a qualified one closer to home.

A letter to the American Academy of General Practice in Kansas City, Missouri, brought the following response in part:

> We appreciate your interest in obtaining a family doctor who keeps abreast of the latest advances in modern medical care.
>
> As Dr. Walter C. Alvarez noted in his recent column, all members of the American Academy of General Practice fulfill this requirement through a program of continuing study. It is the obligation of each member to complete 150 hours of study through scientific meetings, seminars and university medical courses every three years for re-election to membership.

Through the list of qualified physicians in our area, enclosed in the letter, we found a new family physician in whom we have the greatest confidence. He keeps up on new developments, preaches what he practices (and vice versa) and can get pretty "salty" with patients who do not respect their physical "machines" enough to take good care of them. Like most conscientious physicians, he gets as much or more satisfaction from keeping them well as he does from "making them well."

We all know the hazards of speeding. And still we continue to do it and kill ourselves by the thousands each year. We know the hazards of smoking. And still more people are said to be smoking today than before the warning was required on all cigarette packages. We know the hazards of overeating and underexercising and we continue to do both. We know the hazards involved in doing a score of *other obvious* things that can endanger health and life; but because it is human nature to resist giving up that which pleases us or eases our way, we persist, feeling that the disaster will always happen to "the other guy."

Because of this stubborn perversity to act against our own best interests, the problem of educating consumers to use caution even with the most carefully controlled drugs, cosmetics and foods is enormous, frustrating and some skeptics think well-nigh impossible. If, as authors, we let ourselves sink into such skepticism, we would not have written this work.

It is not cynical to say that "people will never learn," for not all people will or can learn because of indifference or inability. But if some people learn about the hazards involved in OTC and prescription drugs, those will be lives protected if not saved.

It is not cynical to say that "pharmaceutical houses don't give a damn about the ultimate safety of their products or the honesty of the claims they make for their effectiveness," because there will always be some companies whose sole concern is "the fast buck." But new laws can educate them in the folly of that philosophy, perhaps not before they've actually gotten on the market with questionable products, but certainly soon afterward.

With the certification of new drugs now demanded under the amended law, the possibility for such abuses will be limited. Even a cynical, dollar-oriented exploiter of human misery in the drug field will come to see that "honesty is the best fiscal policy," morality aside.

In order to better understand the public's attitudes toward drugs, the FDA recently initiated a number of studies. From these it is hoped that a basic consumer-drug profile can be developed that will not only influence the nature of the regulations needed to increase the effectiveness of the FDA's protective measures but may also be useful in determining the most effective educational approaches. Realizing, as it does, that the only way most people can be assured of adequate health protection and maintenance is through the *reasonable use of safe OTC drugs to supplement* the necessary professional visits that one should make periodically, the FDA is diligently pursuing these studies.* The findings will be reflected in drug formulations, directions and labeling and in the general information about them disseminated through the nation's communications media.

Because "Pre-Medicated Murder?" is a service-oriented book, not another exposé that cries havoc but offers few if any solutions, and because of the demonstrated common sense need to attend to many of our minor injuries and ailments without running off to the already overworked doctor, it seems wise in these pages to pass along some suggestions made by physician friends whose counsel we respect.

One of those suggestions holds that every home should have a complete medical guide and encyclopedia. Several excellent ones are available and the inclusion of those mentioned here does not imply that others may not be as useful.

The ones the authors have looked at personally are "The New Illustrated Medical and Health Encyclopedia" edited by Morris Fishbein, M.D.; the "Better Homes and Garden Family Medical Guide" prepared by thirty prominent physicians, surgeons and specialists in every field of medicine, under the editorial supervision of Donald G. Cooley,** and "The Medicine Show," revised edition, a Consumers Union

---

*The *Efficacy of Self-Medication,* Vol. 4 "Philosophy And Technology of Drug Assessment," The Smithsonian Institution.

**The names are a coincidence; as far as we know, Donald Cooley is not a relative.

Publication principally put together in its present form by two distinguished physicians, Harold Aaron, M.D., and Marvin M. Lipman, M.D. Among other honors and positions, Dr. Aaron is chairman of the editorial board of *The Medical Letter* and Dr. Lipman is Associate in Medicine at Columbia-University College of Physicians and Surgeons.

A unanimous suggestion from the authors' local medical consultants requires a dependable first-aid manual in every home. The *Reader's Digest* publishes an excellent one as does the American Red Cross. And "The Medicine Show" contains an interesting chapter, "How To Stock a Medicine Chest."

One is struck by the changes in medication and procedures in some first-aid manuals. Many of the old standby medications now seem to be omitted. Among them are mercurochrome, merthiolate, tincture of iodine, aromatic spirits of ammonia, some proprietary burn ointments containing surface anesthetics and antiseptics, cough syrups and elixirs and boric acid in solutions and powders, among others. Not all the manuals agree and it seems wise, where there is a question, to consult the family doctor or pharmacist. (It is the authors' opinion that the latter's expert knowledge is not called upon often enough by most of us.)

An interesting suggestion and one that seems to make great common sense (although it requires unusual self-discipline) is to keep a monthly family health log. This necessitates a simple notebook or small loose-leaf binder in which are recorded the dates and kinds of vaccinations, any special allergies to foods or medications, the types of self-medication taken and, very important if several doctors are visited, the kinds of ethical medicines prescribed and for what purpose. It is also wise to keep a record of family colds and other minor ailments for which OTC drugs may have been used.

Two doctors said they thought it an excellent idea to keep at hand a copy of the American Medical Association's booklet, *When to Call or See Your Physician.*

All the physicians emphasized the need for periodic physical examinations at least once a year for mature adults

Such examinations should include:

1. A complete medical history including any X-rays that might have been taken previous to becoming a patient of the examining physician.

2. Blood test, including tests for blood sugar, cholesterol and triglycerides; and tests for blood uric acid in order to check kidney functions.

3. Urine specimen.

4. Tests for liver function.

5. For the female, a pelvic examination including a Pap test for those over 35 years of age (routine for all women at Planned Parenthood Clinics) and a thorough examination of the breasts. (Most physicians give instructions for monthly self-breast examinations.)

6. For the male, a prostate examination, including a check of the testicles.

7. Chest X-rays.

8. Rectal examination, including a sigmoidoscopic examination of the lower bowel.

9. Stool specimen.

10. An electrocardiogram for each family member over 40.

11. Basal metabolism.

12. A thorough eye examination.

13. A dental examination.

It hardly seems necessary to add that the regular dental examination and the eye examinations are best done by dentists and ophthamologists. Very often people think that the optometrist who examines their eyes for glasses is, in fact, making a "medical" examination at the same time. Not so, unless he or she is a qualified medical doctor. In one's middle years, it is very important to start having your eye pressure checked for signs of glaucoma, one of the nation's most prevalent blinding diseases.

All the physicians agree with Dr. Walter Alvarez's counsel that the physician should give the patient a "good sizing up," which means that in addition to the tests, the doctor should note such things as height; weight; color and texture of skin; the depth of normal breathing; the size of the liver

and spleen; the "feel" of the abdomen for tumors or rup-
tures; a check of the legs for varicose veins or a possible cur-
vature of the spine; a check of the neck, the armpits and the
groin for the size of lymph nodes; and a check of the
patient's reflexes—with that little rubber "hammer." And, of
course, a blood pressure check.

A great deal of simple, down-to-earth information about
two of our major killers, cancer and heart disease, is available through local chapters of The American Cancer Society and the American Heart Association.

Cancer Detection Clinics in principal cities offer expert
examinations by physicians who volunteer their time generously. The examinations are thorough and the fees for the
extensive laboratory tests are nominal.

Sufferers from other diseases may call the local founda-
tions or societies associated with their ailment for advice on
choosing qualified doctors in their area and locating hospitals with special facilities that may be required.

Certainly all the foregoing is, or should be, generally
known. But time and time again, the authors have heard stories from physicians about the general lack of knowledge of
the existence of various agencies who, had their counsel
been sought early enough, might have helped terminal
patients in time for successful treatment. And most of those
patients had been "treating" themselves with proprietary or
with ethical drugs "borrowed" from friends who were sure
they all "had the same thing."

While the physicians are doing what they can to educate
their patients, the medical profession is taking steps to properly educate or reeducate its own men and women.

In order to make certain that the medical profession consists of competent and up-to-date physicians, the Committee
of the National Board of Medical Examiners is attempting to
revise and broaden its licensing and certifying system.

The chairman of the committee is Dr. William Mayer, Dean
and Director of the University of Missouri–Columbia School
of Medicine. If he and the committee have their way, future

doctors will be qualified by an easier and more efficient system that will ensure patients the best medical care available.

Doctor Mayer and the committee feel that the whole system of medical education and health care in this country presently lacks what the report calls "public accountability." Part of this stems from the fact that most states grant a physician an unrestricted license to practice after one year of internship—despite the fact that specialty board certification by hospitals, many federal agencies and national professional organizations require from one to five years of intensive training beyond internship.

The committee would like to make requirements uniform in all states. They would achieve this by granting a provisional permit to practice medicine under supervision after the applicant had passed a single qualifying examination from the medical school and had been evaluated by the school's faculty.

A full license to practice would be granted by a state board after the physician had received a specialty board's certification. The committee stated that in the near future doctors would very likely be required to take periodic re-evaluation examinations to determine the level of their professional competence. Reassuring news for the patient.

Assuming a "reasonably normal" physical machine, no physician denied the place proper nutrition occupies in the maintenance of good health. And this is an area in which both physician and patient need to know a great deal more.

In Chapter 13, the authors reported that a majority of the physicians interviewed confessed to "deficiencies" in their knowledge of nutrition. Upon more questioning, most of the older men and women confessed that the basic nutritional principles they had studied in medical school had changed substantially during the intervening years and they recognized the need to do more than follow the excellent nutritional columns in the daily press written by qualified professionals.

Actually, as the authors perused the various domestic and foreign professional medical journals in the University of California's Medical Library on the Irvine campus, the practicing physician's continuing educational problem became clear. Quite literally, reams of material are published and not all of it is consistent in point of view or findings.

Many diet items in general use by Americans are now suspect. Coffee and sugar consumption is suspected of having a direct relationship to the incidence of heart disease and cancer. The cyclamates were a boon at first, then a threat—so much so that they were pulled off the market. Now they seem to have been cleared of most charges. It may be that both coffee and sugar will also be cleared, if used in moderation. Ours is not a moderate society. But it is a responsible society. And among the components of that society, the medical profession, for all the criticism leveled at it because of the "high financial profile" of its more successful private practitioners, is among the most responsible of all.

Too often, the work of dedicated research physicians, physiologists, chemists, pharmacologists, biophysicists and nutritionists is lost on the back pages of the daily press—except in those forward looking papers who maintain skilled medical writers on their editorial staffs to continually survey the field for developments that can make important and often exciting features.

In the medical colleges of a dozen great universities, cadres of white-coated scientists, who could double or treble their incomes in private or industrial practice, spend their lives solving the riddles inherent in the human machine. They work selflessly and tirelessly. "I can't leave this experiment right now. I'll be a little late for dinner." This may be one of the most frequently voiced apologies heard, with the possible exception of remorse over the forgotten birthday or anniversary!

A good example of this professional dedication and sense of responsibility is Dr. Roslyn B. Alfin-Slater, Division Head of the Environmental and Nutritional Section of the School of Public Health at U.C.L.A. in Westwood, California. In October 1973, Dr. Alfin-Slater was voted Woman of the Year by her equally dedicated peers.

In a statement released to the press, Dr. Alfin-Slater is quoted expressing her concern about the public's lack of basic nutritional knowledge:

> I must try to bring knowledge of nutrition to lay groups. One of the big community problems is where do you get good information?
>
> Medical schools don't stress nutrition teaching, and doctors don't have the information. If the people who can do it, don't—the public will get it from unreliable sources at health food stores, popular books, magazines, TV programs and neighbors.

It was more than reassuring to have a distinguished research scientist such as Dr. Alfin-Slater confirm something these investigative reporters have been harping on, particularly in our books dealing with the problem of older people and retirees—and most particularly the problems of those older Americans caught in "The Retirement Trap," one dangerous tooth of which is the nutritional problem posed by fixed incomes versus rising food prices.

Moreover, it was heartening to hear Dr. Alfin-Slater reaffirm the advisability of making nutrition a required subject, starting at the grade school level. New teaching techniques that make effective learning "fun-and-games" could be applied. The possibilities are so exciting in their potential benefits for the oncoming generations that the authors often feel genuine anguish that years do not permit the acquisition of the specialized knowledge that is necessary to become effective teachers in the field. But what a potentially rewarding challenge such a career could be for younger Americans who aspire to teach.

There is an old Spanish proverb, a "refran" they call it, that says, *El que hace lo que no debe, sucédele lo que no crée* (He who does what he should not, has things happen to him that he cannot believe).

To do what one *should not* is *not to do* what one should! Hopefully, without "preaching" (because we feel strongly about the need for common sense precautions and sensible health care after visiting hospitals, clinics, morgues and bereaved families), this book will awaken some readers to the urgency of respecting that most miraculous of mechanisms, the human body, in which is housed the only *indestructible* part of we mortals, the spirit.

Admittedly far from perfect, medical services in this country are still among the best in the world. With our energy and imagination, all we lack is the will to make them far and away the best. That will is displayed in thousands of dedicated physicians, dentists and pharmacists. Neither do we forget those equally dedicated nurses and technicians. But too much of their time is taken up with "undoing" damage caused by patients who erroneously feel that lay advice is cheaper than professional advice, that the advertising claims of products yet to be proved safe are "true" and that well-intentioned but unqualified experts in professional smocks and persuasive counterside manners "know as much as the experts."

In the end, how we end up in the struggle for survival will depend upon how much responsibility we are willing to accept.

All machines wear out in time. Abused machines break down or wear out much sooner. If any of us need more persuasive evidence that too many of us are abusing our bodies, we have only to look at the rising incidence of coronary trouble in women and the totally unacceptable coronary casualty list among men (53 percent of deaths) as a result of not taking proper physical precautions in our social and economic battles.

Small wonder that our society is so dependent on drugs. Doctor Edward Brady, Associate Dean of the University of Southern California's School of Pharmacy, points out that drugs were previously used for crisis and short periods of illness. "Nowadays," he said, "people have come to think of them as the solution for everything that ails them."

The only way we can reduce our unacceptable socioeconomic casualties will be to put a ceiling on the price of competitive success and at the same time pay token respect to our physical machinery and its limitations.

"Theirs, not to reason why, theirs but to do and die," may have been said of the Light Brigade, but surely it should not be said of the "bright brigade" who have both the ability and the means to ask the questions and demand the answers necessary to the maintenance of good health—"for so long as the Good Lord Willeth."

Index